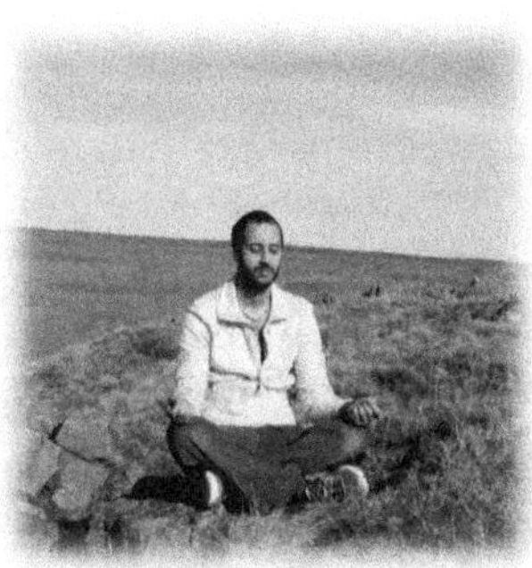

The Fountain of Youth
how to live and feel well

by
W. M. Aslam
2018 © Revised 2020 ©

edited
by
Julie Haley

Sculpture: *The Triangle of Life* created by W. M. Aslam & Mustafa
El-Jarrah, Blyth Beach, England, summer 2015.
Above photograph taken in the Yorkshire Dales National Park.
End of book photograph taken on the River Wear, Durham.

Contents

The Motivation

'Poor diet is a factor in one in five deaths around the world, according to the most comprehensive study ever carried out on the subject.'

-The Guardian Online, 2018.

The Institute of Health Metrics and Evaluation at the University of Washington, America, carried out the study reported on by The Guardian newspaper. So is it possible to eat your way to good health and wellbeing? I believe it is, which is why I have written and published this book you are now reading. I initially decided to compile this book after having observed many people that I know personally who suffer from ill health. They are not old, some are only in their thirties or early forties, but their poor health would suggest that they were in their sixties or even seventies. Their ailments include high blood pressure, diabetes, strokes, poor eyesight, obesity, poor levels of cardio and stamina, backaches, neck pain, obesity, etc. These are worrying signs indeed.

In my opinion, a poor diet and a lack of exercise will inevitably lead to poor health at a relatively young age. Illnesses such as diabetes and high blood pressure were not common among most of our grandparent's generation, and if they were, they would have come about at a much later stage of life.

It is my belief that our current mass consumer age is literally killing us. The burden upon our health and social services is also buckling an already struggling system. Mental health illnesses are also on the increase.

Our mental health services cannot cope with the increasing number of stressed out and drugged up patients. Our so-called 'modern living' has become 'mental surviving' and too many can't cope.

Why is this happening in our so-called 'Age of Information'? What kind of civilization are we creating for the next generation? It is time to reverse this spiral of physical and mental decline. If you are reading this book, you are in a position to save yourself and those close to you from a decline in overall wellbeing.

In this book I include information on how to boost your immune system, digestive system, levels of fitness and energy, increasing strength, maintaining body weight, tips on how to lose weight, increasing muscle mass and toning up, increasing brain function, lifting your mood, improving memory, improving sleep, maintaining good skin, taking steps to prevent illnesses such as diabetes and heart disease, reducing mental fatigue and stress, taking care of your sexual health, as well as other useful physical and mental wellbeing tips. I personally practice all of the advice that I am about to share with you.

On a cautionary note: If you are taking any medication you must speak to your doctor before making any changes to your lifestyle or diet. You should not stop taking any medication given to you for high blood pressure, etc. Best to be safe.

My advice is generic and ideally meant for everyone, regardless of your current level of health. I am confident that after following my advice, you too will soon be living and feeling well. So, let's begin!

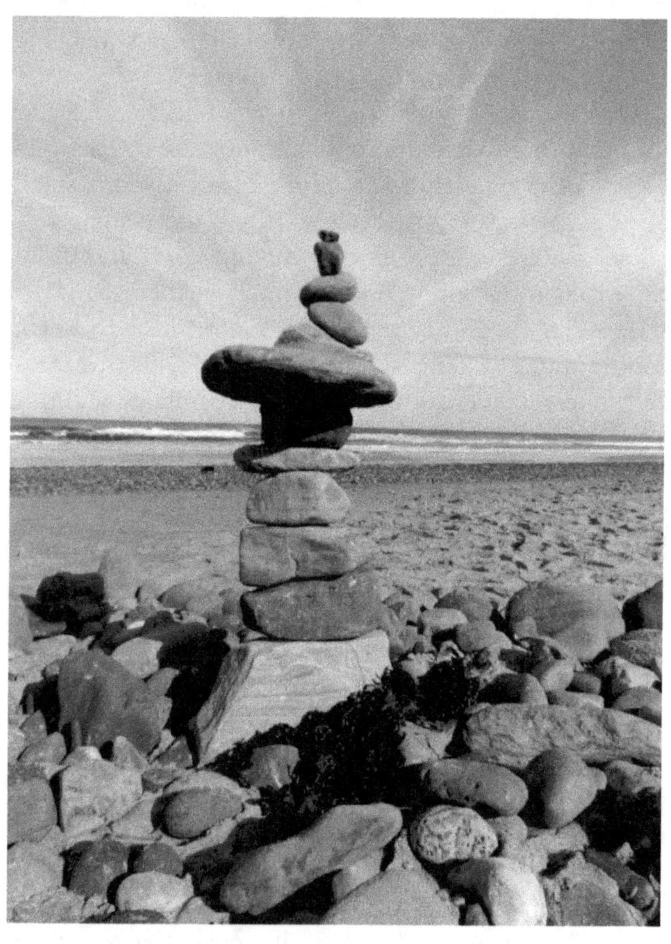

The Triangle of Life (Blyth, England, 2015)

Chapter 1
Me, myself and I

I think I should introduce myself first. I am Waseem Aslam and I reside in the north of England. I will be your guide throughout this book. I have a background in chef work, driving, Art, teaching, acting and writing. I studied Art at college and English language and literature at university. I have travelled in the Middle East, Europe and the Indian sub-continent. I have had the privilege of knowing people from many parts of the world and have benefitted from them both emotionally and spiritually. Living in a very diverse community means I am able to discover many old and new health practices that can both help and heal emotional, as well as physical scars. Our bodies are not machines, they need to be well cared for, and our souls need to be maintained not by drugs, but by holistic and natural remedies. Having benefitted from such natural remedies myself I now wish to share them with a wider audience, with you.

So what made me decide to write this book? This is a very good question on which to begin. I am a forty-three year old male, five feet six inches in height, with a full head of hair and full set of teeth, all my own. I am slim, active, in excellent health and consider myself to be smart. In appearance I look in my early thirties, but am often told that I look in my late twenties. I am reluctant to tell people my real age, they looking so much older than myself. When younger people ask me my age they are always shocked when I tell them I am aged forty-three, and will often not believe me.

I have acted in many television commercials playing age ranges from mid-twenties up to late thirties, my looks being so convincing both on and off screen. My youthful looks did not come about purely by chance however, as I have been interested in health and wellbeing since I was at school, having had role models such as Arnold Schwarzenegger and Clint Eastwood, both of whom have aged well despite now being in their senior years. The late Muhammad Ali and Bruce Lee were also big influences on me. My interest in fitness began largely due to watching these men on television and in film.

I am often told that I must have found the mythical 'Fountain of Youth', which I always find amusing. Of course there is no *actual* fountain of youth, but I do believe that there is a 'fountain of mind'. This 'metaphorical' fountain, like any fountain, needs to be provided with a clean water source, and maintenance in one way or another. In this book I will share with you my own secrets of both feeling well and living well. I will show you how to create your own fountain of youth so that you too can remain active and youthful.

You are unique and you matter because you are here, just as I do. Like me, you too are human, and we are all made of the same elements, and this is why I believe that what works for me will also work for you. However, it will take your own determination and commitment to see the results you desire.

Each chapter of this book contains simple, easy to apply daily routines, which will soon have you feeling and living a whole lot better. You will not have to make any drastic changes to your life, nor buy any expensive equipment or food, in fact, if you follow my advice you will probably end up saving money, money that you can spend on treating yourself. Oh! and do not worry; you will not end up becoming a reclusive spiritual guru, isolated from the wider everyday world. The knowledge I am going to share with you can be adapted to suit stay at home parents to those in high flying careers. So, are you ready? Great!

Chapter 02
Meditation

Okay, I said you would not need to become a recluse or hide out in some remote cave, and I meant it. You may have already heard about the benefits of meditation, well, I am going to tell you about how it benefits me, and that it does not need to take up much of your time. Hopefully you will want to try it too.

My routine begins at around seven o'clock each morning, but yours can begin at any time of the day. I find dawn or anytime just before sunrise a great time to meditate. I will get out of bed, not have any breakfast, but drink a little water, and put the heating on if it is cold. Once my room is at a comfortable temperature I will sit down on the floor cross-legged, and make myself relaxed. If you have a wooden floor you might want to put a blanket or rug down, my floors are carpeted so they are pretty well cushioned. After a few moments of slow breathing I will close my eyes and begin to relax. I will breathe through my nose, as this helps slow down breathing and calm the mind as well as the body. I keep my eyes closed and soon my body begins to feel a mild numbness, a bit like having what we call here in England 'pins and needles'. Soon my lower body becomes motionless.

After about five to ten minutes I begin to enter a mild sleep like state, though I remain fully aware of my surroundings. I begin to think about a place; somewhere I would like to be at that moment, usually a rainforest or a desert. Most days I will end up in a dark and remote location such as a cave or some woods. This is probably the trickiest area of meditation so it helps if you have a picture of the place you would like to 'visit' during your meditative experience. Keep some real pictures to hand that you like, such as those found in holiday brochures, this should help you imagine 'being' there. I enjoy viewing wonderful images online or taking my own, usually of landscapes and skies. Have a look online for such images yourself.

I have been fortunate in that I have experienced vivid visions during my meditative moments, some have been bordering on the surreal. On one occasion I felt that I had disappeared from my room and entered some trance like state in which matter and non-matter had fused together. Then there was the time I felt as though I had shrunk to the size of an ant. Yes, it can get very deep once you begin your journey of mind exploration. Do not fear this however, as you are in control and your experiences will differ to mine.

So try to get some 'Me' time and take five to ten minutes each day to clear out your mind. Try to stop thinking about what is going on in your life, even if for just a short while. You owe it to your mind and body. You will see the results after a few days, and weeks later you will feel like a completely different person. There is really no need to read up on meditation unless it is something you want to explore and delve into deeper, which I think is great. I was introduced to meditation through a friend and then taught myself. It *really* isn't that difficult but books *are* very helpful.

We are all different in how we respond to and utilize the knowledge we are given. There are many meditation websites and articles online that can help you begin your own daily routine. If you search for 'mindfulness' meditation you will find a great deal of reading material. There may even be meditation classes being run in your area. I hope meditation brings you inner and outer peace just as it has done for me.

Chapter 03
Friendships and Relationships

Okay, this is the bottom line as far as this area is concerned: "If anyone messes with my friends and family – they are out of my life." I mean this too.

Why do I focus on friends and family? Well, because if *they* go, much of *me* will go too. No one, and I mean *no one*, is going to mess around with my friends and family. I ask you to take my advice and do the same. Preserve and protect your relationships, as they have taken you years to build but can be destroyed in a day. Sadly there are a lot of jealous people out there.

Now there are probably some of you reading this and thinking that I am being too serious, but I would disagree, just ask the people who are currently drinking or smoking themselves to an early grave after having put up with their so-called friends and family playing mind games on them or worse, interfering and ruining their lives. Family can become your enemy too.

I am speaking from personal experience and a great deal of observation. I come from a family that has a big extension of relatives, both on my mother and father's side. Some of my extended relatives have always interfered and messed around with people's minds, and ruined their lives in the process. Personal relationships, marriages, friendships, all ruined due to their actions, and their victims still feel that they must remain loyal to such people. Suffer fools gladly?

I do not care if it is your father, uncle or cousin giving you a hard time, you tell them to quit messing with your mind, with your life, or you will never speak to them again. No one has the right to interfere in your life, unless you are still just a kid, in which case you will have to wait until you are old enough to speak up for yourself. No wonder many children run away from home. What other choice do they have?

I have had friends for over two years who I have discovered were not really friends after all, and they are no longer in my life. I am not saying not to trust anyone, as you only know if someone can be trusted by trusting them. If they turn out to be untrustworthy, just drop them. That is right; just let them go, for good. I have got some loyalty to family, sure, but I do not go around asking to be slapped on the other cheek. I deal with them on my terms, not theirs. Once trust is broken it is impossible to repair.

So how do I deal with my own friendships and relationships? First of all I make sure I get to know the person well enough to know if they are the real deal. I put down some ground rules, such as no backbiting, no lies, no criticism, etc. You may have your own rules seeing as we are all different. What I am saying here is that you have to value yourself. You do not need anybody to complete you, you are already complete, and that is good enough. Start valuing who you are and be someone that other people respect. They will be grateful for having you in his or her life. Oh, and if you have so-called friends who are drunks and druggies, you should drop them right now, they have got no loyalty to anything but their vice, and when they become an alcoholic or crack head they will be at your door every other day, stealing and lying in order to get their next high.

I enjoy my own company so I am really not desperate for friends. I enjoy various pastimes and also help out in my local community. I find that helping strangers is a great way of filling some of my spare time. I really enjoy networking, and meeting new people who think like me. There is a lot going on locally so go and find out how you can help out. Your input and ideas could change the lives of many people as well as your own.

Chapter 04
No Smoking, Drinking or Lies

Alcohol makes you age, it speeds up the aging process and will leave you looking like you are fifty before you have even reached forty! Alcohol is also the quickest way to gain weight, and the cause of a number of health related problems including liver disease, alcoholism, diabetes, and cancer. Alcohol is the cause of over one-hundred million deaths each year. Here are some shocking statistics on alcohol:

- Alcohol harms are estimated to cost the National Health System (NHS) *around £3.5 billion* annually (United Kingdom figures, 2017).
- 50% of all violent crimes are committed by someone under the influence of alcohol.
- The annual cost of alcohol-related motor vehicle crashes totals more than $44 billion (United States).
- Every day, 28 people in the United States die in motor vehicle crashes that involve an alcohol-impaired driver.
- In 2014, there were 8,697 alcohol-related deaths registered in the United Kingdom, an age-standardized rate of 14.3 deaths per 100,000 population.
- It has been estimated that in a community of 100,000 people each year, 1,000 people will be a victim of *alcohol-related* violent *crime* (United Kingdom).
- Around 50% of marriages end in divorce due to one or both partners' heavy drinking.

You can search online for more detailed information concerning the alarming figures mentioned above. As I mentioned earlier in this book, I used to work in teaching, where over eighty percent of the teaching staff were female. I worked in many different schools, and encountered a lot of stressed out staff, especially in secondary schools. I observed how their nights out took a toll on them, and how they would come in on a Monday morning looking ten years older. A couple of the women I worked with were in their early to late thirties, but an excessive drinking lifestyle whilst at university and then into their teaching careers took a massive toll on their appearance and mental health.

I do not in any way wish to offend anyone, and would never mention any names, but I can assure you that it was common knowledge that some of the staff I worked with had a drink problem. The bottle of wine that was once opened at the weekend was soon opened on a Thursday night, then a Wednesday night, then a Tuesday night, you get the idea. It was not long before wine would be consumed every night!

I can recall on one occasion being asked to pick up a colleague en-route to a staff training day, she was still having breakfast on my knocking at her door, and her breath smelt of alcohol. Alcohol is up there with crack cocaine and marijuana as far as I am concerned. Just because it is legal does not make it any less deadly. Do not make the same mistake as my former colleague, she drove and had two children to look after too! Some of my colleagues pitied her as she was going through a divorce, but that is exactly why she and other women should not drink, as alcohol only provides a short term high, and leaves you with a long term low. Alcohol is a depressant and will only make you more depressed in the long term.

There would usually only be one or two male members of staff at my workplaces, and they tended not to go out much, being more homely types, as were many of the older female teachers that had not grown up in the current 'wine and dine' and 'binge drinking' culture. I am aware that many people drink wine because they believe it to be beneficial. The odd glass of wine is apparently good for the heart. Well, if wine really is good for you, why not try alcohol free wine? It is after all, the wine, and not the alcohol that is said to be of benefit.

I am sceptical when it comes to advice given by doctors. I have known a doctor who used to drink a lot and died of a heart attack in his late fifties. He left behind a young wife, two teenage children, a very expensive house and a prestigious car. Sometimes I can't help but think that a doctor needs a doctor! Have you ever seen a nurse or doctor smoking? I have seen plenty. If they do not care about their own health, why would they care about yours? They are driven by the same desires as every other human. They are not super human; they are flesh and bone, of weak and strong mind like you and me. We need to look after our own health and not rely on the so-called "professionals". Do not forget that it was doctors who were telling the world it was safe to smoke cigarettes back in the 1950s. So what about drinking alcohol? The risk of cancer, whether through smoking cigarettes or alcohol consumption, is exactly the same. This has been scientifically proven. Why are we not being warned of alcohol related cancers? To increase Government tax revenue or maybe to keep the masses sedated?

I do not drink, ever, and this is one of the reasons I look youthful for my age. I look ten; some say fifteen years younger than my actual age. I know my lifestyle has a lot to do with this. Smoking is also an aging agent and should be avoided at all costs, even passive smoking. Bars and clubs are still associated with smoking, even with the current smoking bans in many parts of the world. You will still see people having a cigarette in public spaces, their cars or their homes. Would anyone in his or her right mind sit in a room and set fire to an old car tyre and breathe in the fumes? Certainly not, but this is what smokers do each time they light up. We now know that smoking does not only age an individual, but also kills, as it clearly states on the pack! So why do people who so are obsessed with health and looking youthful risk all by smoking? I think it has a lot to do with the people they hang around with, and the kind of lifestyle they had adopted whilst at school. I know of girls and boys that began drinking and smoking at the age of eight. I have seen it with my own eyes on many occasions. Their parents are often sat in the local bar until late or have no idea what their children are up to.

A good friend of mine is a doctor, and he is always telling me about the trouble alcohol causes in society and to the individual's health. He has had to deal with young women and men whose livers are failing them due to their alcohol consumption, and these men and women are only in their early thirties! What kind of life is that? I spoke to a nurse on one occasion who told me about a twenty-eight year old man who had died from his alcohol addiction. What a waste of a life.

I used to work as a bus driver from 2000 to 2002. The workforce, as you would expect, was largely male. We had two female drivers however. During my time as a bus driver I observed a lot of bad driving, and I suspect, some 'drink driving'. There was one instance that happened to me that I will never forget. It was 11 p.m. and I was driving back to the bus depot. I was about to drive over a roundabout just before entering the bus depot when a small, green vehicle shot past in front of me. Unable to stop the bus in time I hit the car side on, sending it spinning out of control. That's what usually happens when a ten tonne bus collides with a one tonne car. Fortunately, no one was injured, and a colleague of mine who was also driving his bus back to the depot witnessed the accident. The male car driver admitted responsibility, as did his female passenger. His car had been dented but there was no damage done to the bus. I had to call the Depot Manager however to take a formal statement, in case the driver tried to sue for compensation. It was only after the Depot Manager had spoken to the driver that he informed me he could smell alcohol on the driver's breath. I then realized why the driver was so quick to admit being in the wrong and wanting to leave the scene. He did not want the police to be called. This is just one drink-driving incident out of hundreds of thousands. Let me tell you something far more shocking. During my two years of bus driving, six bus drivers were fired for being over the drink-driving limit! You see, it's an addiction, they can't help themselves, and they have no problem with putting themselves and the general public in danger. They don't care about the dangers posed by a ten tonne vehicle. Thank God random drug and alcohol tests are now mandatory for bus drivers, and I suspect lorry drivers too. Imagine how many are never caught? I personally think the drink-driving limit is the problem; all drink driving should be banned completely. People will always assume that they are safe to drive. A total ban on drink driving is the only solution.

Not smoking and not drinking really are 'no brainers' for me, and I hope you will also see that these two habits not only age you, but will ultimately kill you sooner than you think. Of course there is always the 'wise guy' that says things like: 'Well you could get run over by a car tomorrow.' Well sure, buddy, but I have more chance of avoiding that car if I am fit and not panting for breath when crossing the street. I would also like to live an active life and be able to walk to the shops and play with my children each day. Do not keep any 'You could die at any time' people in your life, as you will end up becoming a pessimist just like them. Live healthily and hope for a long life.

It is well known that girls smoke in order to prevent weight gain. This is very common in high schools, but girls as young as ten now smoke regularly. Young girls are full of insecurities, especially with regard to their appearance. They will sooner risk their health than put on weight. Why do they feel so much pressure to look a certain way? The media and peer pressure are the two biggest influences on teenagers. You will find a direct link between a teenager's behaviour by looking at their friends and what they watch on TV, music they listen to and movies they watch. Celebrity culture is another big influence. If you want your children to be free of such influences, spend time with them and help them choose what to watch and who to avoid. I've seen too many nice kids end up in abusive relationships, with criminal records and even in jail.

Lies. Why lies? Well, because lies eat at your heart and soul like maggots devour a dead corpse. My apologies for the gross analogy, but that is how I see it. If you are in the habit of lying you need to end it now. Your heart will suffer spiritually, and you will age quicker with all of those lies eating away at your insides. I am not saying do not ever lie, sometimes we have to, to save a life or save ourselves from something harmful, but to make lying a casual thing and part of your personality is just going to send you to an early grave. Deceiving others will leave you with many regrets, and eventually the guilt will eat away at you. Lies ruin marriages, friendships and societies.

Lying and cheating has become part of the modern world and trust is becoming increasingly rare. How often do you hear of fraud or someone being burgled? What about lying and cheating partners? Hardly a day goes by without hearing about some bad news. I think this is why I rarely watch the news, it's usually full of doom and gloom.

We can all help reverse this trend and feel the better for it. The truth really can set you free.

Chapter 05
Writing Poetry

This is one of my favourite means for keeping an active mind and making sure that I feel good too. Poetry can be enjoyed whether you are writing it for yourself or reading that of other poets. I will attempt to encourage you to write poetry in the form of rhyme and free verse. Hopefully you will find great pleasure in doing so. It really is a wonderful form of expression.

First of all, if you have people around you who think you are crazy for even trying this, move away from them for a while. I want you to be at ease and not feel embarrassed in any shape or form; this includes those of you who already write poetry.

Poetry comes from deep within the heart and mind, from deep within a place where your thoughts and observations linger until they are ready to express themselves. Over time, these thoughts will want to come out, but you will not know how to express them, and this my friends, is where poetry takes over. Write poems about yourself and to yourself, listen to your inner voice and let it soar free of the constraints that you have placed upon yourself. I will demonstrate how I do it, and I want you to try the same activity.

I am sat at my desk at this moment in time, in my comfortable chair, and I can hear the rain falling outside. It is a cold December evening and I am grateful to be indoors and warm. I am going to think about these two aspects, cold December rain, and being warm indoors. From these subjects I will write a short piece of poetry below: -

December, December

December, December
Do you remember -
When I was just a child
The weather being mild?
I would play amongst your cold wet rains
My friends and I would play for days
Upon your pools of melted snow
Running and shouting - our faces aglow.
December, December -
Now I remember
All the delights you had brought
Never feeling a bitter thought
Now I sit here at my desk and write
About those days that just might -
Come back again to warm us all
Come back to warm our weary souls.

I hope you enjoyed this poem; it has brought back fond memories from my childhood, and a more 'innocent' time. This poem took me less than ten minutes to write, and as you can see; it has not been overly mulled over or edited. This is my raw expression inspired by a month and the current weather. I will not claim that you can write this quickly, but after reading a few books of poetry and experimenting with some rhyme schemes, you too will soon pick it up and just go with the flow. I can find some great books of poetry in my local library. I visit once or twice a week. I love to read poems by other poets, they inspire me and help me choose a subject or topic on which to write. So far I have written over fifty poems and have gained a great amount of pleasure from this interest, as well as keep my mind sharp.

Poetry is a great way of maintaining your mental health. I encourage you to not only write poems, but if possible, to perform them too. Performance poetry classes are held in many localities, or you can start your own poetry club. I think it is a great way of seeing the world in a whole new light, and a means to express your thoughts and feelings to a wider and more diverse audience. Poetry is both a performance and a therapy, so try it out and see the difference it makes in your life.

Chapter 06
Stress and Debt

Stress and debt are probably the two most important subjects of this book and which have the greatest impact on our life and health.

I never borrow money that I do not have, simply because it leads to stress when I have to pay it back. If you do not have money, just beg, yes, I am serious, just beg for a living. I am against begging in principle, but if someone really is that broke then there is no harm in asking for a handout. Just stay away from banks and loan sharks that are only interested in getting you into debt. Some charge 67% interest. Did you know that the banks do not want you to pay off your debt? They will do all that they can to "help" extend your borrowing terms, and tell you how easy they will make it for you to repay them. The banks are snakes and scorpions who will suck the very life out of you, leaving you homeless, suicidal or in a mental health institution. They will make you a slave to your job for thirty or forty years and cause you to argue with your family, fall out with your friends, and maybe even drink yourself to an early grave.

It sounds grim, and it really is. The word 'mortgage' pretty much sums it up, mortgage is a French word meaning 'death pledge'. That is right, a death pledge. You pay them until you die! Actually, some people die without having paid off their mortgage, they pass on their filthy 'death pledge' to their children. Nice.

I have met a lot of people in their late forties, fifties and even sixties who are riddled with debt, tied to their death pledge. I am going to refer to it as a 'death pledge' from now on, just so you understand how serious this matter is. The people I met were close to depression, insanity and even suicidal. Yes, you have probably heard of such people, but now there are way more than you could possibly imagine. In England alone there are around one hundred thousand homes being repossessed each year, and families' kicked out onto the street, some with young children and babies! You think the dirty 'banksters' care about you and your children? They will send in the bailiffs and won't care if you have just lost your job, or that your wife is ill or expecting a baby. You are out of there! This is brutal banking, baby!

A few years ago I was looking for some new wheels for my car, not a new car, a car I had paid £1400 for in cash. Anyway, I saw an advert in the local newspaper and decided to go and view these wheels that a local guy had for sale. When I arrived he was busy in his garage. He had a nice fancy home, and they were nice well to do people. I was like hey, just here to see the wheels. He greets me and says, "You interested in a motorbike?"

Turns out that this guy had lost his job and was selling everything! His Jaguar had been sold already and now he wanted to sell his motorbike. You see, he had bitten off more than he could chew, as his bike was bought on his credit card, and his car on finance, both ended up burning a big hole in his wallet and bank statement. What I am saying here is do not get yourself into debt in the first place. People who have debts are never happy and live hand to mouth, or at best from week to week. I know people who earn forty thousand a year, yet due to their death pledge or car finance, they can barely afford to warm their home, or take an annual holiday abroad. Why would you want to do this to yourself? This is self-imposed imprisonment of the body. It is financial entrapment by the banks.

I did not care what people thought of my cheap car, because I knew they could only think that way by being in debt to their lenders. I am free to take work or leave it whilst they are tied to their jobs for life. I actually quit my permanent job in 2013 and many of my colleagues were asking me how I was going to manage. I told them I had no debts and some money in the bank. I would find work here and there on a casual basis. I live in a humble home in a decent neighbourhood which some might think was below them, but I believe that great people make a community, and not five hundred thousand pound houses with no soul, no community, and lots of debt.

Stay debt free, Guys, stay free…

Chapter 07
Water Is Wellness

It is time to turn it down a little and relax in this chapter. Listen, you moisture your plants with water, so why not do the same to your body? I have never heard of anyone water his or her plants with coke, lemonade or chocolate milkshake. You know your body is seventy percent water so give it what it needs. It really is as simple as this.

I quit fizzy drinks many years ago, though I may still enjoy one every month if I am eating out, which is rare. I know people who have fizzy drinks daily, people that are younger than me, overweight, and who get out of breath just walking. Yes, out of breath just walking to the shops or going up some stairs! What is going on with people who drink two litres of fizzy drink every day? Such people will end up killing themselves or ending up with diabetes or other health complications. You do not need all that drink and all that sugar. There are six to twelve spoonfuls of sugar in a single can of coke. This is not 'good' sugar either; it is manufactured and 'artificial' sugar. It is not good for your skin, for your body or for your bones. It is good for nothing, of zero nutritional value. Fizzy drinks do clean rust and sink stains however. Imagine what they do to your stomach?

My daily routine involves drinking plenty of water. I have it for breakfast with my toast, for lunch with my vegetable or meat dish and for my supper. Water is a part of every meal I consume. Water keeps my skin, muscles and organs in good shape. I know you hear some people say, 'Drink four to eight glasses a day', or others might say 'four to eight litres', but the amount is not so important, what is important is that you drink water regularly throughout the day and remove fizzy drinks from your diet.

There is not much more I can add here so I hope I have stressed the point hard enough. I hope that you act upon my advice before it is too late. Water is literally 'Life', and promotes longevity of good health.

Chapter 08
Travel Near and Far

Travel near, travel far, but do travel. You do not have to leave your home country; you do not need a lot of money, just travel and go beyond your own neighbourhood. There is so much to see and so many people to meet. You will find kindred spirits in every community, in every town and in every nation. If you know a trader, or someone that has to travel for work, join them for a week or two. You will meet their work contacts, and see more of life in the process.

I have travelled around the north of England, down as far as London and up as far as Glasgow in Scotland. I am a busy guy with limited earnings, but I still like to get away and see new horizons, and meet new people. I have travelled in Asia and the Middle East as well as Europe. I want to see much more of the world. I really hope that I get to travel more in the near future.

So, you are probably wondering how travel keeps you looking young? Well, there are the obvious benefits of travelling, such as being active and enjoying all the new sights, but there is more to it than just the physical benefits. When you travel you leave behind your friends and family, and have to put your trust in strangers. The people at the airport, the staff at your hotel, the locals and the tour guides. You have to trust people and they have to trust you. This forming of relationships is good for you personally and good for everyone else on this planet. When you meet a complete stranger and hand them your baggage or hire a taxi, you are saying, 'I trust you'. We cannot underestimate the value in each of these exchanges of trust, and the benefit it brings both to the wider world and us as individuals. Trust is good for our wellbeing, it alleviates stress, and this in turn keeps us looking and feeling youthful.

Another reason to travel is to help end the stereotypes we have of other people. Admit it; we all have some stereotypical image in our mind of the Indian, the Chinese, the Arab and even the French. Some of our stereotypes may be negative stereotypes. By travelling to *their* nations we can not only end this practice of stereotyping, but also change our image of an American, a Mexican, Canadian and so on in a good way. Television and movies often portray certain people in a bad light, and this can lead to mistrust of the 'other'. We need to help stop spreading misinformation of others. Free yourself from the mainstream media and political elite and begin to trust again. You will benefit in the long term.

As you travel you are not only expanding your mind, but your very being, by enriching it with a deeper knowledge of humanity. Only a few months back I was travelling in the Middle East when I came across a man giving away free coffee and bread. I asked him if it was a special occasion and he replied, 'No, I just want to share this with you as you are a guest in my city.' I was left humbled. I took the bread and coffee and thanked him before continuing my walk along the pleasant streets.

You see, free of politics, we can all just get along.

Chapter 09
More Lentils and Less Meat

Lentils are life. This is how much importance I give to this simplest of foods. Lentils are a part of my staple diet. They are low in calories but high in nutritional value. They go well with rice, crackers, breads, salads, and even on their own. You can buy lentils in most if not all parts of the world. They are easy to cook; you simply boil them and eat them. Of course you can make great spiced up dishes and soups using lentils too. I also eat them with pasta.

Lentils have an *earthy* taste that you do not find in many other foods, and they come with many health benefits. They can help lower blood cholesterol, as they have high levels of soluble fibre. By lowering cholesterol levels and keeping arteries clean, you can reduce the risks of heart disease and stroke. Lentils also contain folate (also known as B12 and B9), and magnesium, which also helps reduce heart ailments. Magnesium improves blood flow and the flow of oxygen too. Eating lentils can literally give you a happy heart.

Lentils also help with digestion. The insoluble dietary fibre found in lentils can help prevent constipation and irritable bowel syndrome. Your intestines will also need to work less, unlike when having to break down meats that can take several hours to digest.

Lentils can also help stabilize blood sugar levels. The soluble fibre traps carbohydrates, which then slows down digestion and levels out your blood sugar levels. There are many benefits for anyone with diabetes. Lentils also contain a high level of protein. They are a great source of protein if you want to cut down on your meat intake or even go vegetarian. As lentils are slow burning they will give you energy for a longer period of time compared to other foods. They are also a source of iron, which is necessary to provide oxygen throughout your body, and important in keeping the body energised.

If you want to lose weight, lentils are the way to go. They contain no fat but are rich in fibre, minerals, vitamins and protein. They are low in calories but will leave you feeling full.

There are so many reasons to make lentils a part of your staple diet. Give them a try!

Chapter 10
Exercise Every Day

Okay, this one seems really obvious, but most people think of exercise as being demanding and having to join a gym. This is not the case however, and I will prove it to you in this chapter.

I have not been to a gym in over ten years and have no intention to. I own a bike, a mountain bike - but I have never been anywhere near a mountain. I cycle daily, often two or three times a day. They can be short five to ten minute rides, or at weekends a long two to four hour cycle ride with friends, if the weather is mild. I do not cycle in rain, hail or snow, unless it is local.

I actually sold my cherished car over three years ago, not because I was unfit or lazy, but because it was too convenient to travel by car when I could have just set off earlier on foot or by bike. By not having a car I have no choice but to walk, cycle, or run for that bus! I have lost weight, toned up and gotten fitter every day since selling my car. I am now at just less than sixty-nine kilogrammes. I have maintained this weight for over the last two years. My weight at eighteen was the same as it is now. My joints should last a lot longer with a manageable weight to carry and support.

My daily exercise routine begins without breakfast. I drink only water prior to working out and during. I do three sets of eight pull-ups (I have fitted a pull-up bar at home) and follow this by an abdominal workout consisting of:

- Thirty knee crunches
- Thirty cross crunches
- Thirty leg raises
- Thirty cycling cross crunches
- Thirty flutter kicks
- Thirty heel touches
- A sixty-second plank (x2)
- Twenty supermen

Yes, I do have a six-pack. It took me three months to attain. The abdominal area of the body is your core and should be kept well maintained. Your entire body pivots on your abdominals and this is where the support for all of your upper and lower body comes from. Here is a quote from the legendary Bruce Lee on the importance of the abdominal muscles:

"My strength comes from my abdomen. It is the centre of gravity and the source of real power."

Do not lose your core abdominals. Firm up this area. I follow up my abdominal routine with a push up routine consisting of:

- Three sets of ten reps (narrow space)
- Three sets of fifteen reps (wide space)

This workout will give you upper body strength and tone your chest, arms and shoulders. My workout takes me no more than twenty minutes. I will have a thirty second break between all exercises. On top of this I encourage you to walk at least twice a day or cycle, whichever you prefer. My routine is Monday to Friday and I keep to it strictly and so should you. Do not be put off by your age or weight, as it's never too late to get into shape. I know people in their 50s that still run marathons.

If you do not know the moves for any of the workout tips above you can find pictures and videos online. There are lots of motivational workout images and articles so you are sure to find something that suits your lifestyle.

Don't forget to visit your local library too!

Chapter 11
Green Spaces

Green. Go anywhere that is green. Run for the hills! Literally! I try to get out to the countryside at least once a week, even if it is just locally. I am blessed to be living just a forty-minute bike ride away from lush green countryside and about thirty minutes from the coast. I will also take drives out with friends (in their car) but will gladly travel by bus too. My preferred form of travel is always to cycle but it's not always possible due to our unpredictable British weather. Also a good friend of mine is just getting into fitness so an hour cycle ride might prove too much for him this early on. The aim here however is to get to anywhere green. Forests, woodland, country farms, and wild open spaces are just some of your options.

A daily walk in the park can soothe your mind and have a beneficial effect on long-term mental health. Visiting places of nature can have so many benefits that science is still trying to understand them all. It has long been known and accepted that nature is a good thing and that we should do more to interact with our green spaces. Our current generation spends little time amongst nature and too much time on social media, 'liking' beautiful images of sunsets and waterfalls instead of going to 'like' the real thing.

Living in the city and working in a stressful environment can cause anxiety as well as depression. Mental illness is on the increase in our towns and cities, and there does not seem to be a solution to end this trend. There is plenty of research however that shows people visiting green spaces will suffer fewer mental health problems compared to those who do not. We must try to get out to the countryside more.

By visiting parks and woodland we will experience a change in our mood and overall wellbeing. We must start this at a young age and have our children and elders partake in activities such as walking, trekking, rambling or even just enjoying a picnic in a nice park or other outdoor location.

New green horizons will stop you from brooding, thinking over and over again at why your life is where it is and why it had to be this way. To over think can lead to depression so it must be stopped before more serious mental health problems develop. You have to just accept your lot and move on with life, or life will leave you behind.

Get out and get green!

Chapter 12
Reading Rejuvenates

I read as well as write. This can be anything from a post on Facebook, a tweet on Twitter, or a complete novel. Reading has so many benefits and not just for those wanting to further their study and career. If you are not one of those who read daily you could be missing a trick that will give you longevity of the brain. In this chapter I will outline my own daily reading routines and the benefits of reading.

I read one book each month minimum, even if I find the book of no interest. What is important is that I read something. I will always gain something from having read. Research has shown that reading keeps the brain mentally stimulated and can slow down or even prevent Alzheimer's and Dementia. By keeping our brain engaged we could keep it at its optimum power, just like when you keep your computer running instead of putting in on 'standby' or 'sleep' mode.

Reading also helps deal with stress. The modern workplace is not conducive to our wellbeing, unless of course you are one of those fortunate enough to be in a job that you truly love and cannot see yourself ever leaving. The majority of people however do suffer from stress at work to some degree. Losing oneself in a good book helps reduce stress levels and even remove the stress altogether.

Books offer us a form of escapism, so read them frequently. The more you read the more you will learn. A book by a motivational speaker, or someone you admire, will help you acquire new life skills, helping you to tackle any new challenges you may have to face at work or in your personal life.

Reading will increase your word bank too, thus improving your vocabulary and speech. The art of conversation is an acquired skill so you should work on this no matter what your age or occupation. Everyone still loves to talk. Conversation is great for self-esteem and can even give your career a boost. Interpersonal and communication skills are the wires that keep our networks connected.

Reading will also aid your memory, as you have to remember the names of characters, places and events. This is a great way to improve your short-term memory; you will never have to be told an instruction twice or write down that shopping list! You can also do some critical evaluation of the story, plot, and try to figure out the possible outcomes for each of the characters. This takes a great deal of critical thinking and foresight. You can also have some interesting debates and discussions with fans of the books you read. You could even start a local book club!

I am aware that reading is not for everyone, however you can begin by reading 15-20 minutes per day, or a few pages and then work your way up to an hour or chapter per day. Reading is like riding a bike; once you 'get it' you do not want to stop. I recommend a book of short stories to begin with from different genres. Plays and poems are good too, as they do not need so much time to read. I recently started reading William Shakespeare's *Hamlet* and *As You Like It.* These are plays I would never have read in my teens but which I can now appreciate. Reading such texts has improved my own writing too, and given me lots of story ideas for future books.

Books give me great inspiration and a sense of peace and tranquillity. I know that whatever is written in the fictional world of a book is under control. I trust the writer to take me through a great journey and safely carry me to the end of the story. Of course you could read spiritual books to gain the same sense of calm and contentment. Reading in general has been proven to calm the mind, and it is a great way to help us relax after a hard day at work. Watching television however, is a one-way process; you're not mentally active but rather watching passively. You risk becoming a couch potato too. Reading is far more beneficial for the mind.

Visit your local library and see what catches your eye, or have a look online and read some book reviews of the latest best sellers. Make reading a part of your daily routine, you will soon reap the rewards, and share your new-found love of books with others. I know from personal experience that many have benefitted from my reading and knowledge. You will improve your life and the lives of those around you with books.

Books are brilliant!

Chapter 13
Walk or Ride

A walk a day keeps the doctor away, or was it an apple a day? I would say it is both. A walk to the shops or your local park is as beneficial as joining the gym. Walking has been proven to be the best form of exercise that can be maintained throughout a lifetime, unlike running a marathon, or going to the gym, both of which are not possible for many of us. I see many people in their late forties or early fifties walking in my local park due to having been advised by their doctor, prior to this advice being given, fitness was not something they ever thought about. I also advise you to begin walking regularly in your early thirties if you do not already, do not put off exercising until you have health problems and have no other choice.

"When I was anxious and depressed, cycling put me on the road to happiness."
- Charles Graham-Dixon

The above quote by freelance journalist, Charles Graham-Dixon, is just one of thousands of cycling quotes. I cycle every day, even if it is just a five or ten minute ride. Cycling helps maintain body weight, de-stress and regulate blood pressure. It will help keep away many illnesses too, from diabetes to high blood pressure. Cycling has many physical and mental health benefits. Seeing new places is balm to the soul. I often cycle to the coast, about a forty-minute cycle ride, or I will put my foldaway bike on the train, it taking just five minutes by rail, and then cycle along the coast roads. Cycling improves my mood (not that I am ever grumpy) it just means I have a more positive outlook on life no matter what my present circumstances. I meet people wherever I go, and this social aspect increases my sense of well being, *we* being social creatures after all. I feel that my creativity also increases, I come up with more story ideas on seeing the people I meet or the events I observe, conversations I overhear, etc. These all add to my 'Ideas Box' as I like to call it. I usually carry a note pad or will dictate new ideas into my phone and work on these ideas at a later date.

Cycling keeps me in shape, maintaining my figure, and yes, it is important for men too, they also want to fit into their favourite jeans. You can gain a lot of upper body strength and a good posture by cycling just fifteen minutes each day, and eventually gain a flat stomach. If you can cycle without having to use your bike seat this will help you tone up your abdominals, shoulders and arms. Your legs will naturally tone up over time too.

Both walking and cycling I have found help me maintain a regular digestive system and keep my immune system strong. Cycling helps improve gastric mobility in people of all ages, so if you have children you should encourage them to walk or ride with you. Exercise takes a lot of energy but it gives back even more energy. You will feel more energized in the long term. Think of exercise as a daily service and tune up.

Before I end this chapter let me tell you about a man whose life was *literally* saved by cycling. Frank Bowden was an eighteenth century businessman. He had been working in Hong Kong for most of his life. When he arrived back in England at the age of thirty-eight, he was in very poor health. His doctor told him he had just months to live. Frank refused to accept this however and took up the advice of another doctor who told him: "If you want to save your life, take up cycling." (It's always worth getting a second opinion). Frank took the doctor's advice and within six months he was fit again. He was so pleased with his comeback and the benefits of cycling that he decided to buy the cycling company that had sold him his bike. He renamed the company the Raleigh Cycle Company.

Frank Bowden is credited with bringing cycling to the masses. From 1890 up until the late 1990s Raleigh was the most popular choice of bicycle in England and in many other parts of the world. The cycle that saved Frank's life went on to keep an entire nation fit and healthy.

We really do need more people like Frank.

Chapter 14
Family Time

Have you heard of the saying: 'Families that play together stay together'? Those of us from "traditional" families or the "nuclear" family will understand this saying, and know what it means by such families 'staying together'. So what has changed of late?

We are living in an age of independence where family is no longer as important to us. People leave home at sixteen or eighteen and never return other than to visit occasionally. I know it is a global village, but we must maintain our bond with our biological families and local communities, and not be so caught up in our own 'independent' lives that we forget about our own parents and siblings. There can be some moderation to suit all families.

Being there for one another is very important, it makes such a difference to know that you can call a family member for advice or assistance. I know young couples that have moved to the United Kingdom from places such as Libya, France, Syria, India, Pakistan, Egypt, etc. and they all struggle without an extended family network. Childcare is always tricky, and very expensive. Then there are those times when you fall ill, have relationships issues, need some space, etc. The day-to-day practicalities are hard to juggle for a couple with children. Having family nearby is a great blessing, especially for a newly married couple.

Spending time together as a new family is crucial in helping towards the building of lifelong relationships, both within and outside the family unit. Children are taught how to interact with others and play in a fair and socially acceptable manner. It gives them memories too; memories that they will cherish for a lifetime and help get them through hard times.

I can appreciate that it is not always possible to spend lots of time with our children, but even a couple of hours of quality time after school or work is of great benefit. Ask them how their day at school was and soon they will be asking you how your day at work was, and do not feel that you cannot tell them if it was good or not so good. Children need to know that your world has its challenges too, and that the real world is not an easy place to navigate. They will appreciate having parents who will support them however.

Children who spend time with their parents are less likely to get involved with crime or anti-social behaviour. We only have to look at the correlation between absent parents and young juveniles in the prison system. The statistics are shocking. I am appalled to see so many young men growing up not knowing their biological father, and that their father does not care about them, having moved on and met someone else. This can lead to a lot of behavioural problems both in and outside of school. This is why families are so important. An uncle or grandfather can act as a father figure for the boy or girl if their father is absent. I applaud any single parent, whether male or female, these are not easy times for parents.

Try to have family dinners most evenings, and once your children are teenagers you should insist on at least one or two family dinners each week. This will give you an opportunity to catch up and find out how things are in one another's lives. It is also a good way to offer support, as the whole family can offer suggestions for any issues that may have arisen during the week. It is also good to ask for dinner suggestions and if anyone would like to try cooking the following day or week. Such participation helps lower those stress hormones and raise the 'feel good' factor. Everyone must feel like they are a part of what is going on, even if it is by choosing what to eat for dinner or supper.

Try to go out often, as a whole family, the social interaction and exercise will help keep obesity and mental illness at bay. Children can become socially inept if left indoors too much; they need to be outdoors as much as possible. They say you must walk your dog twice a day for around an hour, so why would you keep your children indoors all day? We are social creatures that need that sense of freedom too. I can recall speaking to a child once at school and asking her what she had done during the summer holidays, this was her reply: 'I went to my cousin's house, the dentist, and shopping.'

She was eight years old, and had had six weeks of summer holidays. What were her parents up to?

Family time also helps raise intellect and academia. Children will talk about their schoolwork and homework will become more interesting as a result. Your taking an interest in both of these areas will boost their confidence and self worth. This can be done through hobbies too, so make sure that they and you have interests outside of work and school. There are many after school clubs, local groups and sports clubs for you to attend together or individually. You could even try setting one up yourself. There is a local model boat club about twenty minutes from my house. It is very popular with adults and children. There are also some skateboarding and BMX facilities.

Finally, and most importantly, as a parent myself who is always learning, I want you to know that you too will improve your parenting skills. There is no set manual or method that works for all parents or all children, so do not worry if you find yourself struggling. Making sure that your children know that you love them is enough to help you get through any challenge.

Above all else, enjoy being a parent!

Chapter 15
Charity Keeps You Cheerful

'Give your money to the poor and ask them to pray for you, their prayers are more likely to be answered.'

Charity comes in many forms, a kind word, the offer of food or a monetary donation, etc. Most of us do give in charity, but many of us do not realise how giving in charity helps us as individuals. Giving money to those in need actually makes us feel better, as well as those that are in need. It is a win-win transaction. Giving money in charity releases dopamine in the brain; literally mimicking other forms of pleasure, such as eating chocolate, going on holiday, etc. This psychological benefit if done over a lifetime will keep you in a content and humble state. Imagine what it feels like to be regularly given a chocolate treat, or a surprise holiday? This is how it feels when you give to charity. You are indirectly treating yourself.

There is no shortage of people to help, just look in your own neighbourhood and you will find many victims of the cold, corporate world. Millions of people are seen as nothing but fuel and gears of an economic machine. They have been forgotten by society, becoming outcasts in their own communities. The number of homeless is increasing due to Interest Based Capitalism. Repossession of homes increases year on year, the burden of debt being too great for those struggling the most.

We can no longer rely on our leaders who serve the banks, corporations and weapons manufacturers. Those in need rely on the charity of everyday folks like you and me.

If you see a homeless person and you want to help, try to get them to a project that can offer them help and support, but if they are not willing to go then give them hot food, healthy drinks, fruit and clothing, etc. Only give cash to homeless charities. Do not let a homeless person stay in your own home, your heart is in the right place but you should never let a stranger into your house, especially if you are a single woman or have children. If you know them personally as a friend then of course it would be fine. There are professional organisations and charities to help the homeless, places you can volunteer at too.

No one chooses to be homeless or to live on the streets. By interacting with people in need you will see the reality of this world and how difficult it has become to survive in the tough economic conditions of the 21st century. I am shocked at how many children are living in poverty in first world countries such as England and America. I read in one of the national newspapers that 120,000 children would be homeless in December 2017. This is appalling. Millions are being left to fend for themselves with no help from the state. It is always the most vulnerable that suffer the most.

We need to encourage our own children to give in charity too, that way they will also grow up to become charitable. Encourage your friends and family to donate together, or set up a food bank where those in need or on low incomes can come and get free food. Tinned goods, pasta and rice are always in demand by low-income families. Homeless people rely more on instant hot food or donations of money to homeless shelters. I personally do not give money to homeless people, as there are too many criminals now operating professional begging gangs. I will give money to a local homeless charity, food bank or food kitchen, where the homeless can get food and other help. You should give a homeless person hot drinks and fruit however; even chocolate bars which are not ideal but a good source of energy. I usually ask them if I can buy them a hot drink or some food. It is best to ask in case they have an allergy, or are vegetarian, etc.

If you can volunteer with a homeless charity or deliver food in person (my preferred option) this would be of great benefit to you and those in need. Giving in charity never decreases your wealth; it only increases it, as well as the feel good factor. Homeless people need clothing too, especially in winter. You could give them a winter coat, hat, gloves, even a sleeping bag. Just make sure that any council officials do not see you. Some can fine you for helping them.

If you are one of the fortunate ones who have a secure income, home and family, you have much to be grateful for. I know it is still not an easy life however, as even those with an income struggle and worry about the future in terms of paying their bills or providing an education for their children. Now imagine what life must be like for those that are poor and homeless?

According to many studies looking at charitable giving, donations have decreased over the last ten years. This will be in part due to the financial collapse of 2007-2008. Many people lost their jobs or their incomes were affected, many took a drop in wages in order to keep their jobs. The economic downturn had an indirect effect on the amount of money people donated to charities. Of course the banks are largely to blame for this situation as well as our war mongering politicians. Capitalism only serves the few at the top.

I can understand why some people will choose to donate less to a local or international charity, however, I cannot stress enough that people continue to donate, even if it is less than they would normally. There are not only benefits to those in need but for those who give. Donating money activates pleasure centres in the brain, and can keep depression at bay, something that during an economic downturn is vital in keeping us mentally strong and healthy.

There are always people out there in need, whether in need of food, water or medical aid. They may need some repairs done on their slum home, or even the shack they have built out of waste materials. There is never a 'good' time to donate, as donations are always required, more so in times of economic hardship. With a hike in interest rates and inflation rises we all feel the pinch, our money, no matter how much we have, still seems insufficient for our needs. We can overcome this however by looking at our lifestyle and at what we 'need' and what we 'want'. If we remove some of the 'wants' we can adjust to the economic changes. This will mean that we can still spare some money for charitable causes. You can also get a tax deduction so that the charities you donate to can claim back tax payments using your donations as a taxpayer, often up to 25% in most cases. Donating to charity is a good way of sending less money to the tax office and more to those who really need it.

By donating money to good causes you get to meet new people who think just like you. There will be many kindred spirits out there waiting to meet you. Your combined actions will have a huge impact on the lives of those less fortunate. In the process you will feel a great sense of purpose and gain a rewarding outcome for all involved.

Charity is not all about money, it is also about listening and just helping out in any way you can. One thing I will caution you on however is that you do not end up becoming a 'free' employee. Try to work at grass roots level, with those charities that are free of £100,000 salary CEOs. I am a little cynical, as I know many charities and NGOs use poor people to attract money, both from the private and public sector. I give my donations and time to those charities that pledge 100% to those who are in need. There is no middle management or CEO being paid a whopping salary. Do your research before making any donations.

If you have children it is important that they see or hear about the charity work you are involved with. When they see you being charitable they are likely to follow in your footsteps. I have worked with children in many schools and can tell you that they have a lot of empathy towards the poor, especially if they are also children. During the Indonesian Tsunami appeal of 2004 the school at which I worked raised over £2000. This amount was raised from a school of just 460 pupils. Imagine what those children could achieve as adults? Children do not like to see others suffer and are naturally inclined to give, even if it means they themselves go without. As adults we must never lose this empathy that was abundant in us as children.

If we involve our friends and family we can double our donations. I know some people feel shy asking for charitable donations, but we can always drop a leaflet through doors and people can donate if they wish to. I would never pressure anyone to donate, unlike the big charities nowadays that have sales people calling you up at all hours of the day, and stopping you in the street. These are usually the big CEO charities. They use a sales pitch similar to those of car salesmen or Internet providers. I always tell them I am not interested. I can think of many other charities that will put my money to better use.

You do not need to donate a huge sum of money to make a difference. In the developing world things are still relatively cheap. Vaccinations and antibiotics cost a few pounds. Food and water is less than half the price of what we pay in the West. A little money still goes a long way. Even £1 will help a child eat for a day, or help a baby with diarrhoea receive medical treatment. I am sure most of us can spare £1 per month or give that £12 each year. It will not make any difference to our lives but could save someone else's.

One more thing I would like to mention before I end this chapter concerns gambling, or rather lottery tickets.

People often tell me that they give to charity by way of purchasing lottery tickets. They tell me that a lot of the money from lottery ticket sales go to charity. In England, a meagre five pence from every pound goes to charity. This shows how the lottery creators use the poor and those in need as a means of making millions for themselves. Do not fall for this trap and give your pound or dollar to those in need and not those in greed. The lottery is just glitzy gambling.

The lottery is a tax on the poor and the chances of you winning are slim to nil. Look at past lottery winners and you will see how their lives changed for the worse. Many lost their health, friends, marriages, etc. Money is not the key to happiness, do not be fooled by this lottery business, it is simply another form of gambling. The only way to become rich and successful is by working hard. People will respect you for it too, unlike with winning on the lottery.

Please keep donating to charity, as it will keep people alive and you feeling mentally well and physically healthy. Our world will become a fairer and more prosperous place too.

Chapter 16
Fasting for Fitness

Okay, do not worry; I am not going to ask you to starve yourself. There is a lot more to fasting than just giving up food and drink. There is a lot of evidence that supports fasting as part of a healthy lifestyle. I fast throughout the year, even if it is just water only fasting on certain days. My meals are small anyway so I do not suffer too much from the pangs of hunger.

The best way to begin fasting is to first decrease the amount of food you eat on a day-to-day basis. Decrease your portions of food and then move on to fasting from sunrise until sunset, or if that is too difficult at first, try from 09:00 until 15:00. You can then increase the time from 08:00 until 17:00. This done on Thursdays and Mondays will help detoxify your body, as well as help maintain your body weight. This occurs due to the body being given more time to burn fat cells effectively unlike with a normal diet. Fasting will allow your body to use its own source of energy instead of sugar. Insulin also becomes of effective use due to fasting, which will help keep diabetes at bay. Fasting also speeds up metabolism meaning your body weight will not suddenly increase or decrease. It also improves the digestive system, helping metabolize food and burn off body fat. This in turn leads to healthy bowel function.

It is well known that fasting was prescribed in many faiths, from Judaism, Christianity to Islam. It is no wonder that fasting is still popular in the Middle East, and among the numerous religious communities of the world. There are many spiritual benefits to fasting that you can find out about through your own research. Fasting slows down the process of aging too. If you want to maintain a youthful body and appearance then fasting is the most effective means of achieving this. All of the world's anti-aging creams could never compete with fasting as an anti-aging treatment.

If we look at the larger creation on this planet we will observe animals that eat when they are hungry. Now ask yourself, when was the last time you were hungry? I mean *really* hungry? We eat for pleasure most of the time, and see food as a product. I used to work as a chef so I know about cooking and eating for pleasure, and I also know how unhealthy it can be. If you eat out too much you soon put on a lot of weight, weight that is almost impossible to lose. Restaurant food is rich in sugar, salt and fat. It is a superfast means of gaining weight. If you want to eat out, make it a weekly or even monthly treat.

As a former Teaching Assistant, I saw a lot of children who ended up becoming obese due to their parents always taking them to fast food outlets or restaurants. I can appreciate parents are busy, but how will they care for their obese and sick children in the future if they fill them with the wrong food today?

I was fortunate in that my parents gave me and my siblings home cooked food and the occasional take out around once a month. Home cooked food is always going to be better than eating from different restaurants and take-outs. I eat three times a day. I have a small breakfast, a modest lunch and light supper at around 19:00. I do not eat anything after this time. I brush my teeth and that is me done until the following morning. I try to eat at fixed times too, this helps maintain a regular digestive system.

Fasting helps with brain function, as it increases the production of a protein used for brain activity. I will not go into the science part as it is very complex, but basically fasting can protect your brain from Alzheimer's and Parkinson's disease. Fasting also improves the immune system by reducing free radicals within the body. This can starve cancer cells stopping their formation. By not eating you are also reducing stress, which can help you fight off an illness or infection.

If you want to experience 'enlightenment' and feel 'connected' to the world you should try fasting. With no food to think about or to digest you can ponder upon life and all creation. You can channel your energy into more spiritual matters instead of feeding your primal desires of hunger and thirst. Your mind and body will be 'lighter', allowing you to connect to spiritual matters, such as those of the heart and the subconscious mind. Fasting will also make you appreciate how fortunate you are to have food to eat and increase your empathy for those who are poor.

Fasting can also help improve your complexion and will save you a lot of money spent on skin treatments and creams. Fasting helps clear up toxins, and helps regulate the functions of organs such as the kidneys and liver. You will also note an increase in energy levels right across your body.

I only ever eat when I am hungry and rarely for pleasure. Most people eat food like it is a product rather than to survive. I am all for enjoying a meal but that is not what food is primarily for. It is to keep us alive and healthy.

Fasting has long been a religious tradition, well known to Buddhists, Yogis, Hindus, Muslims, Jews and Christians. There are centuries of evidence proving that fasting is good for the mind and body, and recent science has affirmed this. Fasting for certain time periods is very beneficial for our health. Fasting is becoming popular for this reason. You will not hear many doctors or health "professionals" in the West recommend fasting, which I believe is due to their being in cahoots with the food and dairy industry. This might sound like a conspiracy, but if you stop and think about it for a moment, the food and health industry both rely on you for their living. If you cut down on eating and you live a healthy life, why would you need to go and see your doctor? Would it not also have an impact on the food and dairy industry? It is about keeping us consuming or 'grazing' like cows, and making us ill means more profits for the ironically named 'health industry', it is more of a 'sickness industry' if you ask me. The pharmaceutical companies use doctors as sales people, and they are literally making a killing out of killing us. I have gone off on a slight tangent here so will get back to fasting.

So, what are the main benefits of fasting? This might seem really obvious, but fasting helps you lose and maintain your body weight. I have been fasting since I was in my early teens; it is something my parents taught me. I have always been slim, never weighed more than 80 kilogrammes and rarely been ill. I put this down to a mainly vegetarian diet and fasting, as well as not smoking or drinking, no use of drugs either. I do not look my age; people think I am ten years younger than my actual age of 43. Often people refuse to believe me. I believe I look young due to fasting. I believe food ages us, just like those miles on a car speedometer and the fuel burnt in a car's engine. Imagine the difference between the engines of a car that had only been driven once a week to that of one driven daily? Food wears away at our internal biological combustion engine just like fuel wears away the engine of a car. Interestingly, a car engine also burns a biological fossil fuel, oil.

Fasting helps the body burn up fat cells as a source of energy, which is why many athletes fast to lower their body fat before a competition. Fasting is far more effective than any weight loss diet. Try to fast on Mondays and Thursdays, or any three days during the month, you will see a big difference in your health and body weight. If you want you could try a 'water only' fast to begin with.

Fasting also helps with insulin sensitivity, which means you can tolerate sugar more than if you did not fast. Fasting for a period of time will help your cells use glucose sugars more effectively. It will also speed up your metabolism. This could explain why I am still slim. I have little or no body fat. I always feel energized, even during periods of fasting. My body is able to digest my food and provide healthy bowel function. Giving the stomach and bowels less to do is always going to be a good thing. You will see this difference in bowel function and metabolic improvement over the coming days and weeks.

Who wants to live a longer life? No one knows how long we will live, but fasting has been proven to aid life longevity. Basically, the less you eat the longer you could live. This is apparent in nations such as India, Pakistan and many Arab nations. With the influx of foreign fast foods however there has been a surge in ailments including diabetes and heart conditions. Fast food is literally killing people in the East. They are abandoning their long history of eating less and fasting and are now paying the price.

If you want to live longer you need to make sure you work on your health in your youth so you can benefit in old age. I do worry for those obese Asian and Arab children I now see in the East. Many of their nations do not have the health system to cope with a health crisis. It worries me to see obese children and teenagers and what they will have to endure in later life. It is a health crisis waiting to happen. We need to help reverse this obesity crisis.

Aging slows down your metabolism, but while you are young it can be maintained at a regular rate and keep you youthful and slim. You do not want to gain fat that you cannot burn off in later years. The less you eat now the less likely you are to gain weight later.

When was the last time you felt hungry? Most of us probably cannot remember - especially if we live in the affluent West. After seeing people eat like there is no tomorrow in the East, I imagine many in that part of the world cannot recall being hungry either. You would have to find some homeless or generally poor people to know what hunger is. Our bodies however are designed to endure hunger. The human body can get by on very little food. This myth of men and women needing around 2400 calories per day is rubbish. This figure was probably paid for by the food and dairy industry. No one needs 2400 calories per day, unless maybe they are digging for coal or working on an oilrig. 2400 calories will only make you fat. Drinking alcohol will make you fatter still. It is the main cause of weight gain among both men and women. The 'beer belly' and 'middle age' spread now occurs in people during their mid-twenties! Quit the alcohol!

If you eat a meal every four to six hours you can feel real hunger. I will eat breakfast and then eat lunch four hours later. I will eat supper five to six hours later. I do not eat anything after 19:00. You should never go to bed right after eating. You will put on pounds! If you want to feel really hungry, do not eat for twelve hours. You will awaken a part of your body that tells you to eat to survive, instead of eating out of desire and for pleasure. I only eat when I am hungry. Those days that I do eat for pleasure are very rare, and tend to be on special occasions. If I visit a friend I will tell them in advance not to cook any food and that I will only come for tea. This means less work for my host too.

Fasting helps to regulate our hormones which is how we can tell if we are hungry. Obese people do not receive the signal telling them they are 'full', so they continue to eat until they are sick. They end up with poor eating patterns and often experience major health problems in their early teens and into adult life.

If you never feel hungry you should do something about this. You may need to see a nurse or doctor.

I just want to mention one more thing here before ending this chapter. I am very suspicious of doctors who so readily give out anti-depressants or other medicines to their patients when non-drug alternatives are available. I know they get their commission from the pharmaceutical companies and that this is often their motivation for prescribing drugs. Always do your research and get a second opinion before agreeing to take a course of drugs, especially if they are for any mental health issues. Capitalism has sadly taken over our health system. It is now profit before people.

Chapter 17
Honey Is A Healer

Honey, thanks to bees and plants, has been around for millions of years. It is a natural sweetener that has been known to humanity for thousands of years, the ancient Egyptians believed it had properties to lengthen life and even used it to embalm their dead. A jar of raw honey will remain edible for up to three thousand years! There must be something quite extraordinary about this substance. I think of it as edible gold! It really should be in every household.

Honey helps reduce the risk of cancer and heart disease as it contains many antioxidants. It can help prevent and cure ulcers as well as benefit the digestive processes. Honey is anti-bacterial and anti-fungal. It has been used to treat cuts, minor injuries and infections. Such practices are well known in the developing world and only recently have the benefits been applied to Western medicine. Honey also increases physical performance. The ancient Greeks knew this, as their athletes would eat raw honey to give them more energy. If you want to maintain your glycogen levels you need to replace your sugar intake with natural honey. Be careful when sourcing your honey, as there are many so-called 'pure honey' products that are actually seventy percent sugar. Try to buy from a farmer's market or a trusted supplier.

Honey is added to many 'over the counter' medicines but you can make your own to treat that cough or cold. A single dose of honey is more effective than any over the counter medicine. Giving a young child **(note: <u>do</u> <u>not</u> give honey to children that are under one year old)** a teaspoon of honey before going to bed will help them sleep better too. I have quit sugar and only ever use honey on my cereal, toast, and in my tea.

Honey has been used in Indian culture for thousands of years. It helps promote the natural balance of the body in material terms. It improves eyesight, improves breathing, helps reduce weight and prevents bowel discomfort. It can cure many ailments and infections too. If you make the change from artificial sweeteners to honey you will see the benefit within a few months, and over a lifetime gain much in terms of your physical and mental health. Some people think honey is the same as refined sugar; this is not true, as refined and artificial sugars are known to be a major cause of weight gain and diabetes. Honey has antibacterial properties as I mentioned earlier, whereas artificial sugars do not. Honey contains friendly bacteria, which could explain the many benefits of honey consumption on a regular basis. If I am feeling 'under the weather' (which is rare) I reach for a teaspoon of honey.

Honey will also give you better-looking skin, as it moisturizes and nourishes the skin from the inside out. I used to have mild eczema and suffered from hay fever but this has been remedied since I began using honey daily some five years ago. My dry skin days are over now thanks to my consumption of honey. You should try honey before using any creams or medication. It may work for you too.

On a cautionary note, <u>do not</u> cook with honey; it is always best consumed raw. I know there is a debate on whether to cook or not to cook, but honey turns into a hard to digest 'gluey' substance when heated. This makes it very difficult to digest. As a former chef I would advise you never to cook honey. Eat it raw.

Chapter 18
Ginger Jovial

Ginger is a staple part of most Asian diets and common in the East for both cooking and medicinal use. It is excellent for digestion, as well as having other immune boosting benefits. Ginger tea, ginger biscuits and ginger bread are easily found in most supermarkets, which shows the growing popularity of this wonderful food. Ginger is a natural remedy for colds and the flue, and should be used first and not replaced by over the counter medicines.

You can eat fresh ginger to rejuvenate a poor appetite. It makes a great accompaniment with lunch too, which is when the digestive system is at its most productive. This is why it is better to train before lunch and eat well after, usually an hour after a workout. I often workout at 10:30 and will have lunch at around 12:00. Of course you can always workout before breakfast. The best time to do any exercise is between 07:00 and 11:00. This is when your body is most 'awake' and energised.

Eating ginger helps the absorption of essential nutrients so it is worth taking a ginger supplement if you are an active person. You will find breathing easier too, as ginger helps clear the sinuses, very useful if you suffer from pollen during the summer months. If you travel a lot you can dip some ginger into raw honey to prevent travel sickness. This may not work for everyone but it is worth a try. If you suffer from gas you should eat some ginger to help reduce the problem. Eat a little warm ginger to relieve stomach cramps; it is nice if you warm it in some butter or even olive oil. If you have been training and have an inflamed joint, try putting some ginger in your bath to help soak away the pain. You can use a wet towel soaked in warm water and ginger if you prefer. If you have a sore throat, warm up some ginger tea, it is especially good during the colder months. If you are feeling the blues, some ginger in water will give you a boost. It will perk up your energy levels too, so if you are studying try it instead of coffee.

If you enjoy cooking, try adding some ginger to those rice and pasta dishes. You do not need to add much; even a few grams finely chopped will be of benefit. Ginger is used in nearly all curry dishes so there is good reason to try it in your own cooking. If you enjoy making 'smoothies', try some ginger with blended apples, carrots, lemons or oranges. Ginger cake is delicious too, so try making your own, or just add it to some carrot cake. There are just so many good reasons to add ginger to your diet.

Chapter 19
Garlic Is Great

For many centuries, garlic has been known to benefit the body, even going back to the ancient Roman and Greek civilisations. Garlic is equally a medicine as well as a food. It belongs to the onion, shallot and leek variety. It is very popular in many parts of the world due to its taste and smell. The main use however, just like ginger, has been for its health benefits.

Garlic is very nutritious but has little calories. It contains vitamin B6 as well as manganese and selenium. These are important nutrients that aid general wellbeing. Garlic is known to boost the immune system and can reduce the number of colds and flues by as much as half. Cold symptoms are also reduced by a daily intake of garlic. If you want to spend fewer days on the sick you need to take some garlic as soon as you feel a cold coming on.

Garlic helps reduce blood pressure. It helps lower cholesterol levels. Heart diseases, heart attacks and strokes can be fatal, so use garlic as part of your daily diet to help reduce the risks of heart disease. You do not want to end up on prescription drugs, possibly for the remainder of your life. Prevention is always better than cure.

Garlic contains antioxidants that could prevent Alzheimer's disease and Dementia. Free radicals contribute to aging, but garlic will support your body with protective measures to slow down aging. As stress is lowered by garlic, this in turn will help you look and feel more energized and youthful. The lowering of blood pressure and cholesterol will in turn help you become fitter and healthier.

Garlic consumption is also known to aid brain activity and maintain good memory. You can see this in the chess and domino playing elderly populations across Europe and the Eastern nations such as Turkey and Iraq. Garlic is part of their culinary culture. Garlic could help you live longer too; though it is not possible to prove, but the health benefits are well known. The immune boosting properties and keeping infections at bay are reason enough to eat garlic.

Garlic was once used as a performance enhancing food. It reduces fatigue and helps maintain concentration. It was known to the ancient Greeks, the Olympic athletes were known to use garlic as part of their training diet.

I mentioned earlier that I used to work as a chef. I trained at college and went on to work for a Mexican restaurant and a year later at an Italian's. I am from an Indian and Kashmiri background, and garlic became a part of my diet as soon as I could eat solid food. It was a natural progression to go on to cook Italian food, known for its use of garlic, especially in its pasta dishes. I love to fry onions and prawns in garlic butter, or finely chop some cloves, add to olive oil and spread onto toast. I will use at least three to four cloves of garlic in my pasta or curry sauces.

There are literally hundreds of ways to add garlic to your diet so do give it a try.

Chapter 20
No Takeout

I mentioned takeout food earlier in this book and want to add some more on this subject here. Takeaway food is fast food, and fast food usually means unhealthy food. It is not just the high salt and sugar that is of concern, but also the fact that the food is a new set of ingredients and bacteria for our stomachs to contend with. There is good and bad bacteria, but changes to even good bacteria can present a tough challenge for our body.

Imagine eating home cooking one day, fast food the next, and food from a vending machine the day after? This constant change is not conducive to our body's wellbeing. Our stomach likes to know what to expect, it becomes good at digesting the food we have regularly and when that food changes from day to day it struggles and has to work harder. Think about the times you have been out to eat only to suffer later with stomach pain or just feeling tired or unwell? Different establishments prepare and cook their food in unique ways; they source their food from different parts of the country and even different parts of the world. What about the bacteria from all those hands? Not everyone adheres to a health and hygiene policy, which is why 'open serving' and 'open kitchens' are becoming more popular. Customers want to see their food and how it is being prepared.

I am not saying that you should stop eating out altogether; I am just saying it is better to cook and eat at home, and occasionally eat out, preferably somewhere local.

I see a shift in cooking culture where people will buy the most amazing fitted kitchen but never cook in it! If they do cook it is usually something they put in their microwave or gas oven, ready meals being the staple diet for them and their family. Cooking is becoming a lost skill, beans on toast or fried eggs is pretty much all many can muster. We need to embrace cooking again, as a family, as a hobby, and enjoy the cooking experience together. There is so much more joy in eating food that you have cooked yourself.

Obesity is on the increase, and I do not mean to be politically incorrect here, but when was the last time you saw an obese Chinese kid? What about an obese Japanese kid? Probably never, but I am seeing them now, thanks to the fast food industry and the over consumption of sugar filled drinks.

Just look at the condition of Saudi Arabia, Pakistan, India and Qatar where diabetes and heart disease has become endemic. Over twenty percent of Qataris for example now have diabetes, and in Far Eastern countries such as Malaysia and Singapore the same problem is killing thousands each year. High blood pressure and heart problems are on the increase too.

The countries I have mentioned are places where such diseases were unheard of thirty years ago. An entire generation is growing up on coke, fast food, and sugar filled snacks. I have seen it for myself, men, women and young children all overweight, risking joint pain and breathing difficulties in their forties compared to their parents who may have experienced such health ailments in their seventies. Life expectancy is reducing once more, only this time it is being caused by too much food - not too little. We are not starving to death – we are eating to death.

This is a warning to any of you with children; help them change their lifestyle now before it is too late. I know children and adults like to eat out or enjoy a takeout every now and then, but you must not make it a 'treat' too often, as children especially will find home cooked food 'boring', and eat out more once they start earning their own money as young adults. I see too many overweight young men and women, all eating the wrong kind of food.

Try to live a balanced life using a balanced diet. Too much of one thing is never going to benefit you.

Chapter 21
Cook Your Own Food

When I used to work as a chef I did not eat from the restaurant at which I worked, I preferred to bring my own food to work or chose a healthier option. Do not misunderstand me, Italian and Mexican food, or any other food for that matter, is good, but eating out all the time is not healthy. I am sure there are some great restaurants out there that cook the finest and healthiest of food, but they tend to be expensive.

The foods cooked in most restaurants tend to be high in salt, and though nice to have once or twice a month, are not recommended for daily eating. I know people who eat out two or three times a week, and they have put on a lot of weight. They used to be slim ten years ago but now, and only in their early thirties, have gained around twenty to thirty kilograms of body weight. Men and women who had been slim all their lives have suddenly become overweight. Maybe it is the 'foodie' culture, and the bombardment of dessert parlours now lining our high streets and shopping centres? Whatever it is, it is not healthy, and people are becoming unhealthy due to too much eating out.

I prefer home-cooked food for many reasons, the main reason being that I know exactly what went into my food. I can choose what goes in and what stays out. I know it's healthy. **Eat in, belly in, eat out, belly out!** Remember this next time you feel hungry.

Coming from an Asian background I was raised on home cooked meals, mainly vegetarian, though we would enjoy meat once a week. In my experience, Asian restaurant food, especially Indian food, tends to be the unhealthiest of take-outs. The curries contain far too much oil, fat and salt. I happen to know that salt is added to make customers feel thirsty, that way more drinks can be sold. So the food dehydrates you and then you hydrate yourself (or dehydrate more on alcohol) and then you dehydrate again on the food. This circle of dehydration and hydration messes around with your body's natural ability to hydrate and dehydrate over longer periods of time. The high level of sugar in alcoholic drinks and salt in foods can cause many problems if it becomes part of your lifestyle.

The food industry in general is not at all healthy, whether it be processed foods, fast foods or 'all you can eat buffets'. 'All you can eat' is in of itself spelling out a disastrous unhealthy future. All you can eat means 'pig out until you burst'. This is so irresponsible, but typical of the food industry. You see why I am so cynical? They do not care about our health; they only care about their profits.

I know we all have busy lives and it is not easy to cook every day, especially for a family. Try to begin cooking as a family two or three times a week, you can each take it in turns and suggest meal ideas and who should prepare and who should cook. Someone has to wash up afterwards which in itself can put people off cooking, so choose someone different to wash up each day. There are no dishes to wash at the fast food take-away or restaurant, which is another reason to want to eat out. Washing up is an activity we should embrace however, as it is still a form of exercise. It is better than sitting back and enjoying a dessert or two.

We must try to remain active or we will slow down and become dependent on others and lethargic long before old age. I do not wish to be dependent on other when I am sixty or seventy; I want to be like my grandparents who were active until they passed away.

I hope that you too will strive for a healthy and long life.

Chapter 22
Water – Water

I want to write some more on water, it being so essential for good health and a long life. This may seem obvious, but most people do not drink enough water, thinking that fizzy drinks, soft drinks or just any drink will hydrate them. Water is seen as too 'plain'.

We water our plants with plain water, nothing added, nothing taken away. If it is good enough for plants then it is good enough for us. Could you ever imagine pouring coke or coffee into your plant pot? It sounds ridiculous, but we saturate our own bodies, our 'pots' with all manner of fluids, with the worst being alcohol. Try watering your house plant with Vodka and see how long it lasts before dying? Actually, don't!

Water is the most important component of the human body, it makes up between sixty and seventy percent of our body mass. It varies due to our size but there is no debate on it being the main mass of our body. The earth's surface too is seventy percent water, a coincidence? Regular water intake has many health benefits, plus it is zero calories, and zero fat. Many "experts" claim that eight to ten glasses of water per day will help maintain good health, though personally, I think you could drink less if you were working from home and indoors most of the day. There is such a thing as *too* much water. Sipping water throughout the day works for me, I can drink up to a litre but never more than this. I will have a cup of tea or occasionally a coffee first thing in the morning, but too much caffeine can cause caffeine induced anxiety, and if too much caffeine is drunk too fast it could affect the heart's natural rhythms. Consume caffeine drinks with caution; especially if it is a high-energy drink, which have been known to be fatal in large amounts.

Water keeps us hydrated, just like it does the plant, keeping us both supple and strong. Every cell in our body requires water; so, make sure you maintain your water intake, and visit the bathroom to relieve yourself, as keeping urine within the body is bad for your urinary tract and kidneys. Passing water helps prevent kidney stones, so drink enough water but get rid of it too, do not hold it in. The colour of your urine is an indicator of how hydrated you are, light being very hydrated and yellow being dehydrated. Pay attention to what your bodily fluids are telling you. If you see blood in your urine or stool you must go and see a doctor for advice and perhaps some treatment. Never feel shy to speak to someone about such health issues. There is treatment available and the cure is usually swift.

If you often feel tired it could be that you are not drinking enough water, thus making your body operate less efficiently. It is no excuse saying 'I do not drink much water, as I keep needing to go to the bathroom', this might be an issue you need to take up with your doctor. If you are tired it is usually an indication of dehydration. Less water in the body means the heart has to work faster and get oxygenated blood into the bloodstream. Other organs also become impaired, so do not make them work harder and drink some water.

Drinking water improves overall mood too. With reduced water your cognitive functions slow down, and this in turn impacts on your mood. If you feel a headache coming on it could be due to a lack of water so start drinking, sipping it for five to ten minutes, then make sure to drink throughout the day. Do not gulp water, as this is not good for your stomach or kidneys. As a general rule, one sip for each breath is best. Make sure to sit down when drinking too. This will allow water to enter your stomach gradually. Standing and drinking water can also cause you to choke, especially if you are a young child.

Water is known to help digestion. I find boiled water left at room temperature is best, especially during or after a meal. Warm water helps break down food unlike cold drinks. You can see this by trying to wash your dishes with cold water and then with warm. You will see how the food is broken down with hot water but solidified with the cold. This is what happens to the food in your stomach when warm or cold water is added. Also, if you do not drink enough water it becomes uncomfortable to pass stools, as the colon pulls water from the stools, drying them out and making them harder for you to pass. Drinking water helps regulate your digestive system and maintain hydration so make sure to have it as part of your daily routine. Drinking water also boosts your metabolism and helps prevent stomach pains.

Drinking water before a meal fills your stomach and reduces your appetite, the less you eat the less likely you are to gain weight. We should only eat when we are hungry, so drink water if you feel like a snack. Leave your appetite for lunch or supper and do not snack in between meals. Crisps, chocolate and fizzy drinks are a

, sure way to gaining pounds. By not snacking you will also save your teeth from decay and save money in the process.

Water also helps flush out toxins and gets rid of waste through sweating. This may seem obvious but how many of us really sweat during the day or night? Sweating is a great way of cleaning your skin, so make use of this body feature. A good way to sweat is to jog or visit a sauna. Lying on the beach may cause you to sweat but it's not classed as an exercise, and sunbathing actually ages your skin.

In short, water gives life, and your life depends on it.

Chapter 23
Coconut Catalyst

I first began eating coconut in early childhood when my mother would make desserts using a whole coconut. She would break open the coconut and let me drink the juice inside. She would then cut it into chunks and offer me a piece. I loved the white substance and soon became a lover of all things coconut. There are so many uses for coconut. I will mention some of them in this chapter.

Nowadays there are many foods from chocolate to yoghurt that contain coconut, but I believe the real whole coconut is still the superior product. You can buy whole coconuts from most fruit and vegetable stores as well as large shopping malls.

Coconut provides a quick energy boost, can be used as a hair conditioner, a body scrub, can clean your cutting boards and be used as a lip moisturiser. Give some to your pets too, as it will also benefit them. You can use it in your cooking instead of using oils. It makes a tasty topping for ice cream and cakes. It makes a great natural deodorant. Use coconut oil instead of shaving cream, or add it to your bathtub for a lovely soak to help rejuvenate your mind and body.

You can use coconut oil as a make-up remover; help treat skin conditions and rashes, as well as athlete's foot, ringworm and other fungal infections. Eat some coconut with your food or vitamins to help with mineral absorption. Use it on cuts and bruises to speed up healing. Eating coconut as part of your diet helps with thyroid function. Use it on delicate areas around your eyes to stop them wrinkling. It can be used as a toothpaste or skin lotion and as massage oil. Use on your children's nappies to prevent rashes, use on your own skin to prevent stretch marks. For nursing mothers it is good for increasing milk flow. You can apply it to bee stings and bug bites to heal the wound, eat a spoonful to help with digestion, and help prevent nosebleeds by rubbing coconut oil inside the nasals regularly.

Use coconut oil to help eliminate or reduce headaches and migraines, use as a vapour rub. You can use coconut oil as a leather moisturiser and to polish your pots and pans. Use as an oil for your bike or other mechanical products. Use for reducing heartburn and indigestion problems. Mix with fresh lemon juice and use as a furniture polish. Massage into your nails to heal the roughness and smoothen them out. There are just so many benefits in using to coconut. Have a look online or your local health shop for coconut based creams and oils. For cooking ideas browse your local stores, you'll find lots of coconut based foods and drinks. Be sure to buy some whole coconuts too.

Coconut is really cool!

Chapter 24
Soap and Water

'Cleanliness is half of character and faith.'
-Ancient Arabic proverb

This chapter is on something quite primal, bathing. Yes, we all have to, and *must* bathe. I take great care of my personal hygiene as do most people, and I am careful of the products I use to keep myself clean. I have, as long as I can remember, washed with soap and water, sometimes with only water. Why? Well, firstly, because this is how our ancestors had, until only recently, been bathing for hundreds of thousands of years. Secondly, the bathing products sold in most stores contain dozens of chemicals. If you read the ingredients on the back of a shampoo bottle or any other 'hair and beauty' product you will discover an array of chemicals that you would otherwise go nowhere near.

I know they say chemicals are not harmful in small amounts, but then explain to me why so many men are losing their hair in their early twenties and late thirties? Why is their hair thinning so quickly? I am 43 and still have a full head of black hair, yet I have friends aged 26 to 30 who already have receding hair. My good doctor friend has told me that he also thinks there is a connection between hair loss and shampoos, especially with the use of many different shampoo products. He advised me saying that if I want to use a shampoo I should stick to one brand. He believes the chemicals in many different brands could be the cause of hair loss. He and I have both noticed that people from poorer, developing nations, that cannot afford such products, still retain a full head of hair. They wash with water, and if they can afford it they will use only soap. I have witnessed this for myself, but you can always watch some videos online to see this for yourself. Look at the poor, old men in India, Pakistan or even China. You will see how they have not aged or lost much hair. Indian and Pakistani men are well known for their full head of hair, long moustache and even beards. They retain their black hair for longer too. Here in the United Kingdom I see men with grey and receding hair who have not even reached the age of thirty.

As for the women, I really feel sorry for them. They are pressured into wearing make-up that ages them, they feel they have to dye their hair using chemicals that thins their hair and even makes it fall out. The make-up they apply is full of metals and God knows what else. Many women in their late 20s and early 30s look like they are approaching 50. Then they are told to get a face-lift or some Botox injections. As a parent this really concerns me.

The make-up industries are getting girls as young as seven to apply make-up which is ruining their skin. These young girls want to look older, and the make-up makes them look it too. Make-up ages your skin; it does not do you or your health any good. Make-up is addictive and that is just what the beauty industry want, to make you a make-up customer for life.

My advice is to go back to basics. Use water, and organic soap if you have to. You only need to look at pictures of women from the late 1800s or early 1900s to see how naturally beautiful they were. They remained beautiful until late in life, because they did not have lots of chemical rubbish plastered all over their faces like a layer of cement. They also did not sunbathe, or worse, have our awful sun beds.

Make-up prevents the natural oils in your skin from keeping you looking young. This oil is needed to keep your skin supple and wrinkle free. The make-up industry would have you believe it is better to remove these oils, apply a load of make-up and bleach your hair. This is not only bad for your hair and skin but also bad for your wallet. Make-up and other so-called "beauty" products are not cheap.

I know there is a lot of pressure on men, and especially women to look young. Imagine how your colleagues at work would react if you stopped dying your hair? What if you went to work showing all your grey hair? Would you feel 'old' or 'uncomfortable'? You see how the pressure is created by the beauty industry? Why can a woman not have grey hair? Why should men feel the need to dye their hair? This is a sickness created by an industry that feeds on our insecurities. Look at some pictures of mature men from the late 1800s right up to the 1970s, you will see they have some grey hair, and they were content with it. I have a few grey hairs and I am content. I would never dye my hair; I prefer to remain the way God created me. I am no one's fool or canvas.

If you want to look youthful and wish for longevity, take short showers, use organic soap if you need to, do not spend more than ten minutes showering or you will remove all the natural oils in your skin. You do not need to shower or bathe every day; this is just a marketing ploy by the beauty industry to get you using more of their shower gels and shampoos. Think about it, using their product every day as oppose to every other day means they sell more of their products. I can understand if you have a job working in a very hot environment, coalmine or building site, etc. but anyone with an office job or other admin post should not need to shower every day.

A note for men, grow a beard. Beards have numerous health benefits including preventing skin cancer, keeping skin moisturised, preventing allergies, and prevent bacterial infections. There is a lot of research to back up these claims, I encourage you to do some further research into the benefits of beards.

I grew up in the 1980s and at that time kids would take a bath every few days, some only once a week. Nowadays most children want to shower every day. This is not possible for children in poor households, but look closely and you will see they have good skin. Not bathing every day has its pros. You can of course try this yourself to see if it works for you. I know it does for me.

I will stick to water, free of any chemicals, free of any industrial garbage. You can't improve water.

Chapter 25
Sleep Well

We have all experienced a bad night's sleep. We wake up feeling tired, cranky and even grumpy. We need around six to eight hours of sleep each night. There are long-term side effects of not getting enough sleep; you will suffer mentally as well as physically. There is clear evidence that a lack of sleep presents risks to our long-term health.

Our body needs to recharge itself with sleep, just like it needs food and oxygen to operate. The brain restores its chemical balance during a good night's sleep. A lack of sleep will cause adverse effects upon our brain and body, and prevent it from functioning normally. A lack of sleep can decrease our lifespan too, alarming considering how much time people spend online, often until the early hours of the morning, especially young teenagers. Social media and television networks are available 24/7 and present us with a clear and ever present danger. Many teachers speak of their students arriving to school or college feeling tired, some even falling asleep in class. Yawning, irritability and fatigue are just three signs of a lack of sleep. If you are a student and also working nights you will know how hard it is to focus on your studies, and how hard it is to stay awake during class.

It is no coincidence that coffee is so popular nowadays. A caffeine drink, whether in the form of a cappuccino or high-energy drink, has become the normal means of boosting our tired brains and bodies into action. There have been several deaths linked to caffeine overdose. Internally our organs are being damaged by sleep deprivation. Note that sleep deprivation is also used by agencies such as the CIA and MI6 as a form of torture. It has been used on enemy combatants as well as terror suspects. It is illegal now in most nations but still practiced by many intelligence agencies.

Why is sleep deprivation so dangerous? Firstly, your central nervous system (CNS) relies on sufficient sleep to keep it operating smoothly. Think of your CNS as an information highway, and a lack of sleep as heavy traffic. The flow of information will slow depending on the level of traffic (level of sleep deprivation) and this will have a knock on effect causing your functions to slow down, and the brain will not process information as it ought to. Your memory will also be impaired. It is common knowledge that 'tired driving' is just as dangerous as 'drink driving'. Hundreds of people die each year falling asleep at the wheel. A split second can change lives forever. You will serve a jail sentence if it is proven that you were tired and had fallen asleep at the wheel. This is why truck drivers must take rest stops during their working day and prove that they have had sufficient sleep during the night. Most of us will have seen 'tired' truck driving.

A lack of sleep leaves our mental faculties exhausted and it also ages the body. When you deprive your brain of rest, you force it to shut down itself. These 'shut downs' are known as a 'microsleep'. You will fall asleep for a few seconds, a few seconds that could lead to an injury after a fall or your death if you are behind the wheel of a vehicle. I used to work as a bus driver and saw a lot of road traffic accidents. It was not uncommon to see a car crash on a quiet road with no other vehicles involved. The likely cause would have been that the driver was tired and lost concentration for a few seconds. We have limited control over our brain, if it needs to sleep it will sleep, it does not need our permission. It will shut down whether we like it or not. This is an inbuilt survival mechanism. Do not skip sleep and drive. Get a fifteen-minute power sleep if you are feeling tired, or better still, do not drive at all. We like to think that we are in full control of our body, that there are 'no limits' and that we are 'independent' to the extreme, but this is not the case. Your brain is independent of your body, and when it wants to sleep it will just shut down, regardless of whether you are working, driving, or studying. Your brain will not ask you for your permission to sleep; it will sleep to survive, even if it kills you in the process. Do not drive when you are tired. Your body has its limitations.

I will try to keep things simple and not use too many scientific terms, I am no scientist, and I want to keep you interested whilst you read this chapter.

Our immune system creates infection-fighting chemicals during sleep. We are all familiar with the phrase, 'You just need a good night's sleep'. Sleep is a healer, and the best of healers in my opinion. So many ailments could be cured with the right amount of sleep, and also be prevented with a good sleep routine. If your immune system has lacked sleep you will catch a cold or other bugs more easily. A good sleep pattern will keep your immune system at its optimum 'bug fighting' capacity. Long-term sleep deprivation also poses a risk of diabetes and heart disease. Your health is way too important to throw away on 24/7 entertainments or late nights partying.

None of us want to become overweight, or worse, obese. Sleep deprivation can cause both. Your sleep affects hormone levels and feelings of hunger and fullness. Without sleep your brain cannot tell when your stomach is full or empty, and this can lead to binge eating. This is one of the reasons why so many people snack eat during the day and late into the night. This can over the long-term lead to type 2 Diabetes. Men and women are at risk and it could explain why so many are overweight. Sleep also affects the heart and blood vessels. Sleep repairs blood vessels and the heart. The risk of cardiovascular disease is increased by a lack of sleep. I have a close friend who suffered a stroke at the age of thirty-six. He worked in a stressful environment doing night shifts. He was otherwise a healthy young man. His lack of sleep may also have caused his diabetes too.

Our modern working world is not conducive to our wellbeing. The worst invention in my opinion is the light bulb. All of creation remains within its natural sleep cycle, but humanity is the only creature that works 24/7. The light bulb has many benefits, but personally

I think it has turned us into machines. It is unnatural to work at night. Working under factory strip lights has also been linked to cancer. Night shift workers never see natural daylight. This cannot be a good thing in the long term.

Sleep is necessary in order to produce testosterone. It is very important that children and teenagers get enough sleep in order to have enough testosterone that will help build muscles and help them grow. It is well known that children who suffer from sleep deprivation also go on to suffer physically and mentally. In my opinion, those parents who do nothing to prevent sleep deprivation are abusing their children and should be monitored. The long-term effects can be catastrophic. Allowing young children to watch films and play online games until the early hours is a form of abuse, even if parents think they are giving the child what she or he wants.

I taught at a primary school for over nine years and saw hundreds of children fall asleep during class. They would tell me that they went to bed at 23:00, slept in, and missed breakfast. These children were aged between six and eight. What were the parents thinking? The children's education suffered as a result and yet the parents showed little or no concern.

I cannot stress enough how important it is for us all to maintain a good sleep pattern. You can help your children sleep by turning off the Internet after 20:00 and making sure that they do not use their smartphones at night. The brain needs darkness in order to activate sleep, the light from a phone will prevent this from happening, even if you were to glance at a few text messages during the night, or read an email. The light from the phone screen is enough to kick start your brain activity and you will find it impossible to fall back to sleep. Your mental and physical wellbeing is more important than being online.

Before going to bed put your mobile on silent, place it far away from your bed, and use an alarm clock to wake you up instead.

Chapter 26
Lemons for Life

I have enjoyed the taste of lemon juice for as long as I can remember. I will tell you why you should too.

Lemons are rich in vitamin C and are good for your skin, and can help you look youthful. Lemons rejuvenate your skin from the inside out. They prevent wrinkles and acne. I believe I owe my youthful appearance in part to drinking lemon juice almost daily. I will add a teaspoon of concentrated lemon juice to curries, salads, or to warm water. One glass of lemon juice is a good source of nutrients such as vitamin A, potassium, calcium and pectin fibre. Lemon is also known for its antibacterial properties. Lemon is very popular for its therapeutic uses. It helps maintain the immune system and can help fight off numerous infections. It is no coincidence that lemon is used in many 'over the counter' cold and cough medicines. I can't remember the last time I bought medicine from a chemist. I prefer natural homemade remedies.

Other benefits in drinking lemon water include losing weight and flushing out toxins from the body. It also helps strengthen the liver. By aiding the digestive system it helps prevent constipation, which means no upset stomach to worry about, especially if you are eating out. Lemon water is also very good for the heart and can help break down fats digested during eating. It is also known as an antiseptic and used to clean kitchen work surfaces. The potassium content of lemons also helps nourish nerve and brain cells. It can also help maintain the health of the eyes and can prevent eye problems. A glass of lemon water helps prevent and relieve heartburn. It also helps replenish body salt levels after exercise.

As lemons are acidic they can eat away at tooth enamel. You should only have lemon juice diluted in food and water and rinse your mouth afterwards. This is especially important for children.

Try to make drinking warm lemon water a part of your daily routine. The taste might take some getting used to, but you will enjoy the many health benefits in the long term.

Chapter 27
Fruit Salad

This might seem like general knowledge, but fruit and vegetable salads are a sure way to great health and wellbeing. The water and vitamin content of both fruits and vegetables are reason enough to include them in your daily diet.

Fruit has always been present in our family home and continues to be to this day. There are no chocolate bars or sweets in our home; our 'treats' come in the form of fruits. I feel I owe a lot of my youthful appearance to consuming fruit on a daily basis.

Fruits will benefit your body a great deal as they are rich in vitamins and minerals. These are essential for your body to function at its optimum level. They are also rich in dietary fibre, which helps the digestive system function. Fruits are a good food alternative if you want to lose weight. They will give you enough energy and the nutrients that your body requires to get you through your day. You won't have to worry about any additional fats either. Fruits can also help you avoid heat stroke, cancer, heart ailments and diabetes. Fruits can fight off skin disorders and keep your hair healthy and strong. The best way to benefit from fruits is to eat them raw. This is far better than processed fruits found in drinks or desserts. Try to make fruit a part of your daily diet. It will help you avoid processed foods and preservatives too.

Fruits help boost the immune system, something we can all benefit from in this modern age of stress and long hours at work. You are less likely to become ill with a diet rich in fruit, always a bonus if you tend to suffer from colds or flu. Fruits are also linked to improving mood, something people in colder climates will appreciate, and what with the little sunshine to boost their mood. Fruits also provide a quick energy boost, so try an apple or orange instead of a coffee next time you are feeling lethargic.

Many of us will take multivitamins; I include myself in this group, though I tend to have them every other day, as well as vitamin D due to a lack of sunshine in the winter months. Fruit can provide us with the essential vitamins in their natural form. These natural forms can never be replaced by over the counter supplements. If you do take supplements keep taking them until you can replace them with a natural fruit alternative if possible.

I have been eating fruit and vegetable salads with my meals since I was a young boy, salads being a staple part of the Asian diet. I don't mean the mixed salads you buy in the supermarket here; I mean the home cut salads using fresh produce form local groceries. Cucumbers, onions, lettuce, tomato and olives make up the best part of a good salad in our home. I encourage you to make them a part of your home too.

As for fruit in my home: oranges, pears, apples, grapes, kiwi, plums, bananas, etc. are regularly bought and eaten. You can make them into 'smoothies', enjoy slices with ice-cream, or even have them in between meals. I will make sure to have at least one piece of fruit each day; I don't always stick to five a day.

Eat what you can of fruit and vegetable salad; just be sure to eat some of both every day.

Chapter 28
Up to Date

Dates have been a part of my diet since childhood. They are very popular within Asian and Arab culture and their health benefits have been known for centuries. Some of the benefits include relief from heart pain, diarrhoea, and constipation. There is also research being carried out to show how dates can prevent abdominal cancer.

Dates are rich in vitamins and minerals as well as fibre. They contain magnesium, potassium, calcium, iron and copper, all of which can benefit your health. If you want to maintain a balanced diet you should eat dates daily. Eating three dates a day can keep the doctor away. They are also good for anyone wanting to gain weight, and this is why gym goers and body builders consume dates, either whole or as part of a milk shake. You can create a paste and blend them with yoghurt too. Dates are also known to speed up recovery from any injury and in providing much needed energy. The sugar in dates is far superior to refined sugar. Try to stop using refined sugar and switch to dates instead. Try chopped dates in your tea or with your breakfast cereal.

It is well known that Muslims break their fast with dates or water. The feelings of hunger are soon alleviated thanks to the high nutritional value of dates. The potassium also provides the nervous system with a quick boost. This is very important for anyone who has been fasting all day.

Dates are also linked to good eyesight, and preventing ailments such as night blindness. Many studies have shown that eating dates can help maintain good eye health and overall vision.

Dates are now classed as a superfood, due to their significant amounts of minerals. They are good for strengthening bones and fighting off bone diseases. You should give young children at least one to three dates per day to ensure good bone development, and elderly people should also eat dates to help maintain their weaker bones.

Dates are rich in iron so can treat anaemia. They help increase iron levels within the blood and this leads to more energy and less fatigue over time. You will find that eating dates will make you much more energised whether you are anaemic or not. Try dates instead of coffee, energy drinks or chocolate. The natural sugars like glucose and fructose found in dates are much more efficient and healthier for the body. They make a great snack for when you are at work too. Try keeping some with you next time you go to work or to the gym. You will see how effective they are.

Dates have many health benefits, but do be careful when choosing dates, as their sticky surface can attract bacteria. Make sure you always check the produce, and ideally it should be packed or sealed in plastic. Be sure to wash the dates before consuming them. You don't know how or where the dates were stored before you purchased them. Of course this is a precaution and should be followed even when buying loose fruits or vegetables.

Discover dates for a healthier life!

Chapter 29
Ivory Smile

You only realize the importance of your teeth when you reach your 30s. Hopefully you will not have had a sweet tooth in your youth, or been snacking throughout the day. Visiting the dentist can be painful for your gums, and also for your wallet. A check up will cost you around £18, a polish another £15, a crown a whopping £240! With prices like these you will want to look after your teeth from an early age.

I never had a sweet tooth at school, but I made up for it at college, though I wish I hadn't. Crisps, sweets and fizzy drinks are the staple diet for many school children and young teenagers. I can recall fizzy drinks being banned at two of the primary schools at which I worked. All too often a child's lunch would consist of a packet of crisps, a chocolate bar, and a fizzy drink. As you can well imagine, the children's teeth looked like brown wooden sticks, I exaggerate not. I was so concerned with the poor condition of the children's teeth that I voiced my concerns with both office staff and class teachers. I saw the issue as neglect and even abuse. The sweetest children would feel embarrassed by their decaying teeth, and many were self-conscious. What were the parents thinking? Surely they can teach their children good dental care? I saw many children aged between eight and ten with rotten adult teeth!

The main cause of tooth decay is too much food, any food! We are all aware of the dangers posed by sugary drinks and treats, but eating any food leaves behind food deposits on the teeth that are broken down by bacteria, and the bacteria excrete a by-product in the form of acid. It is this acid that eats away at our tooth enamel.

If you want to keep your teeth in good condition, eat less, and brush between eating. I eat breakfast, brush my teeth, eat lunch, brush my teeth, eat supper, and brush my teeth. You do not always need to use toothpaste; you can use a mouthwash or empty toothbrush. By brushing in between meals you have an excuse not to snack. When I visit a friend or relative and they ask me if I would like some tea or something to eat, I will often tell them that I have just brushed my teeth. Your teeth will last you a lifetime if you practice this too.

I am going to include some other useful tips here that I have discovered during the writing of this book. I will not be going into all of the science behind each health tip, but will mention the benefits I have discovered.

Cranberries contain vitamin C, K and fibre. They can prevent urinary tract infections. They can also help prevent stomach and mouth infections. Men and women experience such infections so I encourage you to use this natural medicine to prevent and help cure any infection.

Kiwi fruit are filled with vitamins C, E, copper, magnesium, potassium and fibre. Kiwi fruit is effective in preventing colds and other infections including respiratory disease. Not to be given to small children however, as it has been known to cause allergies. It also helps lower blood cholesterol and reduces the risk of blood clots. Has also been linked to good vision.

Oranges are rich in vitamins A, B1, C, folate, calcium, potassium and fibre. Oranges contain many disease-fighting properties. They are known for their immune-boosting properties. They help prevent colds and other infections. One medium sized orange is sufficient for the body's daily needs. Oranges can help prevent stomach ulcers and kidney stones, as well as help diabetics control their blood sugar levels.

Raspberries can help prevent yeast infections and irritable bowel syndrome. They also help protect eyesight and in maintaining blood sugar levels.

Brussels sprouts are among my favourite foods. Not only are they delicious, but also contain vitamins B1M, B2M, B6M, C, E, and K. They are rich in carotene, folate, calcium, copper, iron, magnesium, potassium and fibre, as well as omega 3 oils. No wonder my teachers and parents encouraged me to eat them! They are great for supporting the immune system, especially during the colder months. Brussels sprouts are also good for maintaining healthy skin.

Carrots are great for eyesight and overall vision. The nutrients in carrots help you see in bad light. The best way to eat these orange lovelies is to cook or juice them. Try them with other vegetables to create many new carrot rich dishes. I like to eat them raw too.

Onions are one of my favourite and daily vegetables. They have been known for their healing power for many centuries, and make the stock for most Asian curry dishes. Onions help keep diseases at bay so it's worth adding them to your daily diet. I have been eating onions regularly since I was a young boy. My mother got me into eating onions with her homemade salads and I have been a fan ever since. They contain anti-inflammatory ingredients and nutrients that can counter breathing problems and help ward off the common cold. They also contain antibacterial properties that can help combat infectious diseases. They protect the intestines and work with the digestive system to help prevent many diseases. Many people do not like the smell of onions, but it is worth thinking about the benefits to your health instead of what your breath smells like. You can always brush your teeth or chew on some mint leaf afterwards.

Sweet peppers, like onions and carrots, can also help with eyesight and breathing. They can boost your immune system. They contain antioxidants that can counter cell damaging free radicals, as well as protect against the common cold. Rich in vitamin C, they can help reduce eye disease and fight off many diseases. They are a versatile vegetable and can be eaten with many dishes as well as salads.

Coriander is a food ingredient I have been eating since I first began to eat solid food. It is commonly used in hot countries and in hot food. No curry goes without it. It has been used largely to prevent food poisoning in the form of a herb and spice. It contains antibacterial elements that help prevent salmonella and keeps away any bugs. It is used across Asia as a healing remedy in many forms, especially for inflammation. I eat coriander almost daily and encourage you to try it too.

Black Pepper contains potassium, a mineral that helps improve your digestion of food. It also maintains a healthy intestine. It also helps prevent gas. Peppercorns are also known to help break down fat. I use crushed peppercorns on my toast every day.

Mustard was never a part of my early diet. My white English friends introduced me to it. I liked the taste right from the start and still use it in salads and with other savoury snacks such as samosas and pakoras. Mustard contains vitamin B3m, calcium, iron and magnesium. It helps prevent inflammation of the lungs and can improve lung function. If you work around people who smoke it can be of great benefit (though it's best to avoid second hand smoke).

Turmeric is another spice that I have grown up with, it being essential in any curry. It contains vitamin B6, iron, manganese and potassium. The trick with turmeric is not to consume too much. A teaspoon in a curry is more than enough to help prevent many ailments such as bowel diseases and help relieve arthritis pain. It can also help with liver function.

Chickpeas contain folate, copper, iron, manganese, fibre and protein. These really come in use if you work a lot. The minerals help ward off infections. If you are not a big meat eater you should eat chickpeas to maintain your iron levels. Chickpeas also help stabilize blood sugars and help deal with preservatives found in many foods. Chickpeas have long been a favourite food of mine. I encourage you to try them too.

Lemon is one of my favourite ingredients. I add it to curries, fried egg, chicken and even lentils. It is rich in vitamin C and flavenoids. It has cleansing powers and antioxidants. It's great for a detox, as it can suppress the appetite. You can try fasting with a lemon juice only fast. You will also notice how fresh your breath smells. Lemon is known for aiding digestion; hence you get it with kebabs when you order a fast food meal. It can help relieve bloating and heartburn. Lemon helps strengthens the cells in your body so make it a regular addition to your diet.

Apples are great for detox and digestion. They are rich in pectin, fibre, vitamin C and K. They contain life-enhancing nutrients. The main benefits however, are with digestion and detox. Eating an apple will help you feel full and stop you from overeating. This will give your stomach less to do. It can also help prevent constipation, more common nowadays due to unhealthy eating or not eating enough. You must do all you can to prevent constipation as it will prevent your body from getting rid of toxins. The fibre in apples helps food progress through the gut and picks up any toxins. The fibre softens the body's waste so you won't end up with constipation meaning you can pass waste easily.

Apples are known as a health food in many parts of the world. I can still recall being given an apple each day at school. I never understood the nutritional value of fruit back then, but I'm grateful for it today.

An apple a day really can keep the doctor away!

Chapter 30
Final Thoughts

I hope that you have been enjoying this book and my thoughts on wellbeing. I try to make my findings interesting and useful. I will summarise what I have learned so far from my life in this final section.

Our bodies are made up of 70% water. Our bodies *are* the fountains of youth. Within each of us lies the means with which to live a long and healthy life. Our fountains, if given good nutrition, will produce a crop that we can harvest during our lifetime. We must not mix alcohol, nicotine or unhealthy foods with our 'metaphorical' fountain. Our fountain contains everything we need to live a rewarding and healthy life.

With a simple exercise routine we can maintain our body and continue to look and feel well. We have a choice to remain fit or let our body slump into a lazy life of daytime television and medication. We can choose right now how we want to be at sixty or seventy years of age. We can choose to work less, earn just what we need, instead of hoarding our wealth. We can choose to save our sanity by meditating and by removing ourselves from stressful situations. We can choose the friends we want for life, by making sure that we maintain a close circle of friends and maintain our friendships as though they were our family. We can choose what we eat and drink. We can choose to keep our fountain clean and maintain its purity.

One last thing I will mention here concerns vaccinations, or rather vaccinations for children and the elderly. I have two young children, and both were vaccinated. They are doing fine, both in their health and academia. I often have young or new parents tell me about the dangers of vaccines and that they are not sure whether to have their children vaccinated. I can tell you from almost ten years of working with children, speaking to parents and educators, doctors, child psychologists, and my own research that you *should* get your children vaccinated. Vaccines operate on a molecular level, so even if you are religious, vegan, etc. and do not wish to use a product containing animal fat, etc. you need not worry. You are not consuming the actual meat of an animal; it is merely biological chemicals used at a molecular level. It will not harm your body or religiousness.

Please safeguard your children and do not be misled by the scaremonger and conspiracy theorist. There is no proof to my actual knowledge that vaccinations harm people, but I do know that by not vaccinating it will cause millions of deaths. In many parts of the world the Polio Vaccine is not available, especially in remote areas. Thankfully it is now being made available. You can help bring vaccination to remote communities of the world and help children succumbing to Polio, Measles, Hepatitis B, C, Malaria, etc. I have seen the detrimental affects of not vaccinating children. You must have your children protected, especially if you travel abroad. Three of my friends became seriously ill whist working and travelling in Australia, India and Indonesia. None of them had had their vaccinations updated.

Where you go from here is up to you, but I hope that you will take life by the horns and meet every challenge with determination and optimism.

****

Thank you for reading this book. I intend to continue learning, as I believe I have merely touched the surface of 'wellbeing' and have so much more to learn. There is an ancient Arabic proverb that sums up my attitude towards learning and it is this:

'An individual will attain knowledge for their entire life, until finally they will say; 'I have learned everything', after which they will have become ignorant.'

Live long and live young!
****

I have written many online blog posts related to wellbeing. I have chosen some of my favourites and included them in the final pages of this book. I hope they will also benefit you and your loved ones.

The Box

"You need to think outside the box." Our boss, friend, colleague, partner, etc. will often tell us this. We have all heard the expression 'outside the box'. Some of us hear it several times a week. Well, here is something I discovered recently - there is no box! That's right, no - box. There is no room, no ceiling, no walls and no box! We are free to just 'think'.

This 'box', metaphorically speaking, is keeping us locked away, afraid to speak, making us fear our very thoughts and ideas, wanting us to never explore beyond our comfort zone, or to allow anyone 'inside'.

Every box that I know of is good. There is the box we receive gifts in, the phone box we call someone from, the sandwich box we carry our lunch in, the new shoe box, the post box, the soap box and so on. So why do we carry this negatively charged 'box' around all day?

Who gave us this belief that we are trapped inside a box? I think I may know.

This 'box' is not a box; it is a cage, a barbed wire fence, and a mental prison. It is time to escape this mental box, to stop people from telling us to 'think outside of it' when we were never inside it in the first place. Those telling us to 'think outside of the box' are the ones who put us inside there in the first place. We must tell them that this 'box' does not exist and to refrain from using such an expression in the future. People should not assume that we are 'inside' a box. If we continue to propagate this 'box' we will end up boxing in other people too. We will also tell them to think outside of an imaginary box, and thus make them feel trapped or worse, inadequate.

What makes me so passionate and keen to share this with you? It is through my writing, and having had time to think, that I came to see how we as a people could be manipulated into certain ways of thinking, to become, 'institutionalised' for lack of a better term. We are all creative, we are all capable, on a 'cline' or 'scale', but none of us are trapped inside a box like some shelf product with a sell by date. If I cannot think outside of the box am I less worthy than someone who apparently can? No, by no means no. If anyone is going put me inside a box it will be me.

My box has gone, thrown out, in the recycling bin. I am myself and I live in the real world. I still like boxes, only real boxes!

There is no box, there is no box, there is no...

Alone, But Not Lonely

'Endure happiness and sadness yet remain silent.'

Being alone, this is something we must all experience at some point in our lives. There is however much to gain from being alone. Do not worry; none of what I am about to share with you involves sitting in a darkened cave and meditating, though I would certainly not discourage such pursuits.

Thoughts of loneliness and being alone came to me as I wandered the beautiful streets of Paris, and whilst viewing the many wonderful art galleries. I have also recently returned from a trip to the Middle East, where I also pondered over such thoughts, having met many lone travellers who were keen to explore their wider world and mind. Most of the travellers I met had stressful jobs and many responsibilities, and wanted to enjoy some time on their own, not a bad thing, and definitely not selfish as some might see it.

Personally speaking, I have enjoyed my own company, or 'being alone' as some might conclude, for many years. I first enjoyed my own company whilst in early childhood. I would be engrossed in a good book or making plastic kit model cars or aeroplanes. During my college years this progressed to spending many hours studying alone. At the time I was studying Art, it being a favourite subject of mine since I was at primary school. Creating art allowed me to spend a lot of time on my own. Art is such an absorbing and therapeutic activity. I was amazed at how much creative output I experienced during those times of seclusion, and how much more I valued the time I spent with family and friends.

After leaving college, and feeling somewhat disillusioned with Art and the Art Establishment, I decided to work full time in various professions, as well as continue painting on a commercial basis for both friends and corporations. I would often finish work at around nine or ten o'clock on an evening, and then come home to spend several hours painting. I would paint until the early hours, often until dawn. Those were my 'golden hours', a time in which I would find myself most absorbed in my art and being open to inspiration. There are 'windows' of inspiration.

Dawn really is a mysterious and magical time. As a painter creating images on canvas I saw it as a transition between the death of night and the birth of a new day. Many of my favourite artworks were painted during this 'golden time', most of which I went on to sell to private collectors, some paying hundreds of pounds for my work. I guess they saw the same raw, poignant imagery that I had seen during my moments of inspiration. It would be difficult to recreate such art.

My ten-year spell of painting came to an end (temporarily) when I discovered my love of writing. It was during periods of being alone that I also wrote my first novel. I enjoyed the experience so much that I made it a routine to spend time on my own, to enjoy my own company and hope for more inspired stories to reveal themselves. I am now writing my fourteenth book! I have recently experienced another creative period during which I have written three books off poetry that I am very satisfied with. I am now writing a fourth collection.

I believe we should all spend some time alone, to carve and create a personality which others will enjoy. We should read the literature of past writers and notable individuals. This will help us shape the person we are to become. How can other people enjoy our company if we do not enjoy our own? This is a question I often ask myself. I strive to better myself and enjoy who I am before allowing others to enjoy my company. I expect the same of others too.

By spending time alone I can assure you that you will never be lonely. You will always be with your thoughts, words, art or the company of those who value your company. Do enjoy time with yourself.

<u>Don't Remain In The Harbour</u>

Imagine if you had met someone who had never sailed their ship, never flown their plane or never driven their car? What would you think of them? Like me, you would probably feel that their ship, plane or car was being put to waste. More importantly, you would feel that they were missing out on life's adventures. You see, just like ships, boats and other vessels, we too are created for travel and exploration. However, our 'vehicular' bodies carry not passengers but rather our souls and memories. The soul yearns to see new horizons, to experience the salty air of the seas, the lush grassy fields of the countryside and the dry heat of the desert.

Our vessels, though not tied up with mooring ropes or shut behind garage doors, are often bound by the Ropes of Capitalism. That's right, the 'Ropes of Capitalism'. You have seen those ropes too, the 'mortgage ropes' which people tell you to tie around your ankle for thirty or forty years, the 'car finance' ropes, the 'you must get married now' ropes, the 'you must have children now' ropes, the 'you must have a permanent job' ropes, the 'you must go to university ropes' and all manner of other ropes.

I can recall many incidents where people were being advised (or gently pressured) to buy a house, a newer car, seek job promotion, etc. all because the people advising them had done similar things in their own lives. The one I dislike the most, however, is the 'you need to stop dreaming and get a proper job' ropes. I use the plural 'ropes' as there is always more than one person telling us to 'tie' ourselves down.

Now I am not saying that people should not buy a house (without a mortgage of course), get married or have children, what I am saying is that you do not have to jump to people's expectations and orders, but to rather do things when you feel you are ready.

I once overheard a lady be told, 'You are thirty now, you really should find yourself a husband'. The lady being advised felt helpless and was unable to reply, no doubt feeling that the advice she was being given was somehow right. Sorry, but you do not get married because you are thirty or forty, you get married because you have found someone compatible, who loves you as much as you love them. Do not fall under the pressure of others, wait for the right person to come along. The worst thing you can do is to get married under pressure, only to find out later that he or she is the wrong match for you.

You see, this Capitalist mentality of always going for the bigger and apparently "better" thing is leading to people's unhappiness. Why not just be content with what you have? I have seen plenty of people burn out due to a promotion, whereas they were quite comfortable in their previous role. Why should people keep climbing the career ladder, because society expects them to? Why should they tie themselves to a thirty-year mortgage? ('Mortgage' incidentally is a French word that translates as 'death pledge'). You literally pay it back until you die. Trust me, I have seen enough people nearing retirement with one foot in the grave and still paying off their bank mortgage. I once went into my local bank to pay in a cheque and on leaving I was asked by one of the bank employees if I would like to apply for a credit card, here is my transcription of that *very* brief conversation:

Bank Employee: Can I interest you in a credit card, sir?

Me: No, thank you, I don't need one.

Bank Employee: You never know, you might, it is good to have one.

Me: I am very good with my money.

Bank Employee: You get an overdraft limit of £1500, which can come in handy.

Me: I have never overdrawn and don't intend to.

Bank Employee: Okay, sir.

The banking system is to me what Las Vegas is to gamblers; it is a chance, a risk, and a scam. You buy a house for £100,000 and pay them back £200,000. How does that work? Because we 'suckers' and 'fools' make it work. Money does not grow on trees, but it sure grows in banking computers. They make money out of nothing from nothing. Some digits transfer from their account to the buyer's bank account and that is all they have to do to double their money. How can the same bricks and cement be worth double in just one transaction? Then there is the 'negative equity' to worry about. Look at the housing collapse of 2008, especially in Ireland, where people still have mortgages of up to £750,000 with homes now valued at less than £150,000. The banking 'house' always wins just like in Vegas. They trick you into putting those ropes around your ankles by showing you the glitzy world of win, win, win! But you can only lose.

I know a guy who has £7,000 of debt on his credit card and his wife another £11,000. No doubt they both met a very nice bank employee too. People keep telling me there is no alternative to mortgages and loans, but this is because they have had their confidence taken away from them and Capitalism injected into their very being. Stop buying into mortgages and watch how soon the price of houses will be reduced to the value of bricks and cement. If we continue at the current rate we will end up with a super-rich and super-poor. It is already happening in cities such as London and Paris, where an average house costs £500,000. Your university degree will no longer secure you a salary to enable you to buy a house. Even many doctors are in mortgage debt!

Debt can destroy your dreams so stay away from finance, especially credit cards. I know people earning £40,000 a year and they still rack up credit card bills and cannot even afford a yearly holiday. Live within your means, not within your dreams.

Now this may not surprise you, but I would like to remind you of this fact: Banks <u>do not</u> want to help you pay off your debt. They want your debt to last for your entire life. Yes, I know this will not surprise most of you, but it amazes me to see so many people still taking out credit cards, loans and mortgages when they clearly cannot afford to pay them back. Now that most post-graduate students will leave university with a minimum of thirty-five thousand pounds of debt, you can expect things to worsen still.

If you think back to the heyday of industrial England, when individuals left English harbours and set sail around the world, or made great discoveries here at home, you will recall that they were not tied to a lifetime of debt, or that much praised 'job for life'. They were free-spirited individuals that would take off whenever they felt like it. They used what little money they had in their savings to work their way from place to place, often setting up businesses both at home and abroad. Interest Banking has killed this free spiritedness. It keeps us forever at port and in fear of poverty.

Let us just imagine for a moment that we, yes, you and me, are having a conversation. We are both mature people and both have a university education with good jobs and many future prospects. I tell you that I have decided to sell up everything and move to New Zealand to become a shepherd. What would you think of me? Now you may well be fine with the idea and think it is great, or you might think I am crazy to give up a secure job and my comfortable life in England. But what criteria would you be judging me by? Would it be the current Capitalist criteria and social values, or it could be your own sense of what life means to you personally? You see, in my view, a shepherd is just as important as a well to do property developer or luxury car salesman. It is about what you value personally that counts, not what society values. If I were to listen to the people who tell me I am crazy for wanting to become a simple shepherd, I would literally be turning away from my own destiny. We should not let people influence us in this way. We must not let others scare us into thinking that by leaving the harbour we will be at risk from storms and sinking. I may have a Romantic view of the life of a shepherd, but it is my view and that is what is most important. If I can 'see' my dream then I will work hard for it, even if no one else can.

It is important to listen to your heart as well as your mind. I believe we are given both physical as well as emotional signs in life, and these signs guide us toward our real destiny. Along the path to fulfilment we will meet many, maybe even hundreds of negative people, all saying we are crazy, that we will never do it, that it is a waste of time. Remain strong and keep clear of such individuals, they only want to hold you back.

I am sharing these thoughts with you because I have done all of the above and never regretted it (apart from becoming a shepherd which does appeal to me). It is amazing how when you are looking for something someone comes along with that very thing you were seeking. Is it a coincidence or fate? I believe it is all written by the same greater power, known by many names. 'The pen has been lifted and the ink is dry' is an ancient Arabian proverb used to suggest that our destiny has already been written. You need to believe in a path you cannot see but which is definitely there.

When you do finally make a decision, you must realise that it is only the beginning of your journey. Just like diving into a river you will be carried from place to place, not knowing where you might end up, or whom you might meet. The possibilities, however, are endless and unimaginable.

Remaining tied up in the safety of the harbour, and fearing the storms and strangers will only lead to a life unfulfilled. So release those mooring ropes, open up that door, and set out on a journey of self-exploration.

You owe it to both your mind and body.

The Broke Artist

Yes, you read the title correctly, 'The Broke Artist'. Why did I choose this as my title? Because most artists are broke for one reason, they offer to exhibit their work for free. Let me tell you a little story about one artist who used to be broke too, only he undertook a steep learning curve and is now financially stable and actually earning money from his art.

I was a sibling of five children, my father worked as a baker and my mother cared for us full time. We came from a working class background and enjoyed a happy and comfortable life. I had been interested in Art since I was at nursery. I would paint on anything with anything, from leftover emulsion to half empty spray-paint cans. I would make use of anything I found to help me get creative. As any artist will tell you, art materials are very expensive and 'Art' is usually the pastime of well-off individuals. I could not afford to buy new paints and brushes with my pocket money, and had to make do with what little I could buy at car boot sales or from friends. I was very resourceful however and my parents would help me find materials from a variety of places. I would mix my own paints and use cheap paintbrushes of any kind to paint with. From these humble beginnings I discovered my creativity and love of Art. I soon began to paint and decorate our home with my father who also enjoyed this activity. I have lost count how many rooms we have decorated over the years. My real passion however was painting on canvas, and as soon as I left school I went to Art College, where I studied Drawing and Painting, Graphics, Textiles and Photography.

After two years of college, and wanting to experience the world of work, I put off going to university. I decided to work for myself as well as take on several temporary jobs. I soon found some work as a chalkboard artist and began to be paid well for my work. I also began painting on canvas, which I would display and occasionally sell locally. The problem with exhibiting, however, was that no gallery would be willing to pay me for exhibiting my artwork. They would just tell me how much publicity I would get and that I may even sell my work. Well, let me tell you the publicity was not worth it, as I was soon broke. This was a steep learning curve for me and I became somewhat disillusioned with the Art World.

During this period I had also learned that people do not respect artists like other professionals, largely because artists do not respect themselves. Can you think of any other professional who would work for free? Imagine if you asked your local mechanic to come and work on your car for free, and that he would get lots of publicity by working on your drive? He would tell you where to go! What if you asked your local hairdresser for a free haircut, and in return you would tell everyone how great they were as payment? He or she would feel insulted no doubt. So why do people expect artists to come and display their work for free? The reason is this; the artist thinks that they are getting a good deal out of it.

Most people working in galleries, and the general public, seem to think that an artist just comes along and sticks his or her artwork on the wall and then goes home. They also often assume that the artist is rich, what with the £300 price tag on their work. That may be the only piece he or she sells that month or even that year. Artists have rent and bills to pay too!

Dear Artists, let me tell you exactly why you should not work for free. You spend weeks creating the art for the theme of the exhibition, pay for it to be framed, transport it to the venue, spend time liaising with the gallery staff, turn up at the opening event and mingle with organisers and attendees, yet you do not get paid a penny! How can this be right? The fact is no matter how much publicity the gallery receives you still might not sell any work. The gallery however, gets the visitors they wanted, the commission on sales and a free exhibition put on by the artists who fell for the 'free publicity' trap. You see why artists are broke?

So, my message to artists is not to exhibit their work in any gallery unless they get paid. I would not even exhibit my art in the Tate Modern unless I was paid for it. I would want travel expenses covered too. Why should I work for nothing? Pay me or do not bother calling me. I value my work and myself even if others do not. Try getting any other profession to work for free and then you'll know how artists' feel.

Nowadays I tend to do commission work for friends and family. Word of mouth is the best way to promote your work. I also receive referrals from many people and have sold my art nationally.

If you do not wish to be another broke artist I suggest you follow my principle and stick to it. Do not fall for the 'Lots of people will view your work' or 'You will receive lots of publicity' rubbish. Have some self-respect and conviction in your work. Once people realise that artists will not work for free, the galleries will have no choice but to budget for artist fees in their expenses for any future exhibitions. Galleries are usually run as a private business or charity, and both will have a budget for expenses. They should pay their exhibiting artists and stop being greedy. They are a business first and charity second. I hope as an artist you will seek payment from now on, and not feel embarrassed in asking for payment. Just be professional and reasonable with your fees. I once put on an exhibition over a weekend for £150.

Most of all enjoy your creativity regardless of whether people value it or not.

<u>Fifty Shades of Clay</u>

After having watched several videos related to the Donald Trump rallies and the racism inherent in his supporters, I decided to write something on the issue of racism, it still being a huge problem internationally.

Seeing Trump supporters with 'Make America White Again' banners and watching many of them assault people of colour worries me. It shows that America is turning into something very ugly.

Racism post-abolition of slavery has never been addressed. In the 1970s and 80s black musicians and singers, especially from the Hip-Hop community would express their resentment of the police and the institutional racism prevalent in U.S. Law Enforcement. Whether it was the police, FBI, CIA or any other agency, racism was a major factor in the locking up of millions of black Americans. Back then there was never any proof of this racism, unlike today where the killings and beatings of blacks are recorded on camera. Sadly, even with video evidence, white police officers are rarely charged with an offence. Of course not all police officers are racist, but there are a lot of racist officers who are not being charged for their crimes, even when caught on camera. No wonder black people feel alienated and like second-class citizens. Having a black president did not make their lives any better either, the same way a female president would not automatically make women's lives better. The policies do not change due to the gender or colour of a president.

The issue of racism has finally been acknowledged and must now be addressed. Black History (from African origins) must be taught in schools, as well as the shameful practices of slavery and confinement. Yes, there will be horror stories, but just as we have all learned about the horrors of the Holocaust, so too will we eventually come to terms with the horrors of slavery. Hiding history only makes matters worse.

We are made from many shades of earth, from both a scientific viewpoint (carbon) and a religious one (created from clay). The clay found on our planet ranges from white to brown to black, hence a good simile to liken our skin's appearance. Medical science has shown how the blood of a black person can save the life of a white person whose biological family may not have the right blood type. This can also be the case for a white person donating their blood type to a black person, etc. Imagine if a racist individual were offered a kidney or heart from someone of a different colour, would they turn it down and rather die than take the organ? I seriously doubt it.

If we look back at our recent history, we only have to go as far back as 1980s Apartheid South Africa to see just how evil racism is, and the long-term trauma it can cause. Both black and white people have suffered because of racism, although understandably the black indigenous South Africans suffered a great deal more than the white colonizers. Now we see racism rearing its ugly head in places like Israel, Germany and France, where far-right groups and politicians are clamouring for votes. If there is one fact I know about politicians it is that in the last one hundred years they have caused the deaths of over two hundred million people. World War One (caused by the Royal Families of Europe) cost over thirty-eight million lives, World War Two over sixty-million, Vietnam over three-million and Communism over fifty-million. The current 'War on Terror' has cost over five million lives!

Racism has deep roots, which can be traced back to the Greek and Roman civilizations with the persecution of Jews and Africans. Of course more recently we have the persecution of Muslims, and this stems from a European history of religious persecution by the so-called 'religious elite'. Catholicism has had its fair share of dark eras too, such as the Crusades against Muslims and expulsion of all Jews from 15th century Europe. The Jews were given sanctuary and safety in Muslim lands.

Fear is a major cause of racism and politicians know this. They use this primal emotion to rally support for their bigotry and create violent, irrational beings that go on to persecute others. Interestingly, the amount of DNA that makes up the colour of our skin is the same as the amount that makes up the colour of our eyes. Imagine how stupid people would seem if they hated others because they had different coloured eyes to their own? This is exactly how stupid the racist ideology really is. People like Trump and his supporters worship the dollar, fame and celebrity. He will bring anarchy to a new level and America's downfall. He reminds me of a Roman emperor, Caesar perhaps? Or is it The Madness of President Trump?

Racism lies at the root of many wars. The hatred of others, especially foreigners who speak a different language, or those of a different colour can be reason enough to kill. We really must stop our leaders from dividing us further. Why should a Pakistani hate someone from India? Why should an American hate an Arab? Why should the Chinese hate the Japanese, because their leaders tell them to? What kind of stupid reason is this? We need to find ways of cooperating with one another in what is a finite earth with finite resources. I hate to imagine the final death toll if a nuclear war were to break out.

I can understand how people in the past may have felt that we are different 'races', but science has shown that we are only one race. Each of us being different is a blessing, as we can come to recognize and know one another. Imagine if we all looked the same? A child would not be able to recognize his or her own parents and siblings. If we all looked the same life would be so dull. By our appearance we can see who is from which nation or family. Life would be confusing if we all looked alike, and just think how many cases of 'mistaken identity' and fraud there would be? We should be grateful that we are not like certain species of monkeys, birds or cats which all look the same. We are unique in that we are all individually different, even identical twins are not really identical. Be happy being different and celebrate our diversity.

The main purpose of this post is to show how we all matter, and that no matter what you are going through in life, you will find a solution in the end. We need to support one another as a creation and do more to heal past wounds. I see too much fighting and division, used especially by our political elite. It is time to realise our true purpose in life, and that we all matter as much as the next person.

I hope that through my poetry and story writing I can play a small part in helping unite humanity.

The Value of Friendship

A relationship that is often overlooked and not given much importance in this day and age is friendship. In past times, a real friendship was valued as much as a real love, a family member or even a protective guardian. Friends would die for one another; put themselves in danger to protect one another, sacrifice wealth and health for each other.

When I observe people nowadays, especially children, with few loyal, or even shockingly, no loyal friends, I wonder what they have not been taught regarding the value and rules of friendship. I know people in their sixties and seventies who have had the same friends since they were at school or university. I can appreciate the world is changing fast and so will friendships, but I still feel this is an area everyone can and should value more. Friendship should be taught in our homes and schools. We should never underestimate the value of true friendships.

Friendship is a topic I enjoy writing about, whether in my fictional stories or poetry. I was blessed with great friends both at school and right up to university. They were not only great friends emotionally but also very physically protective over me. In return I gave them loyalty and advice like any good friend would. It was through these friendships that I learned about life, and the lives lived by people from other parts of the world, as well as those in my own local neighbourhood. I was gifted with seeing more of humanity and became a better person because of this.

The special friends I have met over the years still to this day influence my writing. I wish I could thank those who for some reason or other drifted away. When life moves on it often takes old friends away too. Work, marriage, children, etc. can mean our priorities change and so will our circle of friends. I remain thankful for all of my former and current friends for the great memories they have given me during my life.

It is upon friendship experiences that I also reflect. In my college days I had a friend who I never truly valued or saw the beauty in. I always kick myself for being such a fool. I guess we drifted apart and lost touch. I still feel a 'soul' connection however, and believe this aspect will always remain with me as a reminder. Sometimes friends come into our lives for a single purpose. I believe that particular friend I lost came to teach me the value of friendship. There should be no regrets.

Friends are our companions just as much as a husband, wife or child. Life, and our very communities are weakened by a lack of loyal and trustworthy friends. We live in a disposable society where friends are dropped like litter and picked up elsewhere like bargains. Why has it come to this?

Maintaining a real friendship takes time and effort, it takes patience and dedication. Friendships need not be high maintenance but do require nurturing and time to maintain, this can be done through mutual agreement to suit all. A true friendship will survive the test of time and distance.

I hope you will always value your friendships.

The Ugly Industry

Yes, you read the title correctly, 'The Ugly Industry', and not the so-called 'Beauty Industry'. If this is all you take from this blog post then you have taken enough to realise that it is largely men who now define "beauty", and not the women it is supposed to benefit. Women are the victims of fashion.

It is men who tell women what constitutes being beautiful. Men that want women to fit their standards of beauty. They put women under enormous pressure to look a certain way. These standards are not fixed either, for example in England, China and India the standards of beauty are very different. What is seen as beautiful in one country might be deemed unattractive in another. I really feel for those women who move from one country to another, only to find that they are no longer considered beautiful. An example might be a black woman moving from her native African country to the West, or a pale white Western woman moving from the north of England to a sunnier Spain, where a tanned complexion is favoured by men. Note that it is men who advise women on beauty, from telling them what they should wear to how they should style their hair. Why did women allow this to happen?

Beauty is in the eye of the beholder; it is far deeper than what is seen on the surface. Personally I find intelligence to be the most attractive feature in a woman. It is my personal choice, which I would never impose on women however; as I am aware that beauty comes in many forms. I find it despicable that men judge women and have the nerve to comment on which woman is the most beautiful at work, in a pub, in a family, etc. Such men are themselves ugly on the inside and are hardly qualified to judge. Beauty pageant events or 'pervert parties' as I refer to them, are for such sick perverted men. This is an area where feminism has failed women and where feminists show their weakness. How come men do not have to wear make up, put on a swimsuit and walk around like a piece of meat? Again these events are run by men, and judged by men. I find them despicable.

Nowadays we see women going under the surgeon's knife as though it were as simple as visiting the dentist. There are so many treatments available that I cannot list them all here, but they include lip injections, tummy tucks, breast implants and fat removal. Then there are the more cosmetic treatments such as eyebrow shaping, nail and hair styling. How come society will not allow women to grow their hair grey yet men can? A grey haired woman is viewed in a negative light and made to feel uncomfortable, but George Clooney is made into a sex symbol. Why the double standards? How come men are not under pressure to do their eyebrows, wear lipstick and foundation? Why the hypocrisy? What kind of equality is this?

The definition of beauty has been warped by the so-called "beauty" industry. I call it the 'ugly industry' because its main purpose is to make all women feel ugly so they then end up buying more products from the sellers of this sick industry. I have read and heard about many women that are actually beautiful by society's standards, yet lack confidence and view their own appearance as being 'unattractive'. Such women idolise the women they see on television, music videos and in celebrity circles. The famous women they admire are either airbrushed in magazines or have had so much cosmetic surgery that it would be impossible for the average women to live up to their standards.

Look at the world's most famous fashion designers and you will find that they are mostly men! I refer to them as 'fashists', as they use advertising more like a fascist regime would in power. They make women feel inadequate and "unfashionable", and this is their main concern. You are "out of fashion" and therefore an outsider, a social outcaste. Children are not spared this awful treatment either, as they are also made to feel worthless, and many will even commit suicide after years of bullying from other school children. You can do an online search and find hundreds of cases of child suicides for yourself. I have worked in education for nearly ten years and have read many of the bullying statistics to know how children are bullied for not wearing the "in" clothes. It is easy to knock the confidence out of children, especially the girls who are full of insecurities before even starting high school. Slim girls see themselves as fat, and skinny girls think they need to diet! Beauty really is a beast.

Again I would like to point out that beauty is subjective. The standards and tastes in beauty change over time. In the 1930s thin women were portrayed as being beautiful, in the 1950s it was the fuller figured woman, in the 1960s it was the thinner woman again, in the 1980s it was the athletic woman, in the 1990s the thinner woman, and now in the 2010s it is the fuller and well-bottomed woman. Note that these trends will be different again in every nation. Look at what the Swedes, French, Germans, etc. found attractive during these eras I mentioned and you will see stark differences in taste.

In the Middle East and Far East, women are again viewed very differently. The one thing they all have in common however is that men define what is beautiful, and not the women who actually reinforce these so called "standards" of beauty. It is as though women are self-hating while they continue to perpetuate the notions of beauty passed down from their men. Such culture is very unhealthy and must be stopped.

Behind all of these images of beauty lies the so-called beauty industry. Their goal is to remove the confidence from women's minds and replace it with anxiety and insecurity. Once they have made women feel worthless without their beauty products they will create repeat customers for life. To counter this propaganda, women need to empower themselves and their bodies must be viewed as sacred. No man or woman should have the right to belittle them or make them feel any less of a woman. Keeping away from reality television and beauty magazines are very good ways of maintaining your own self-confidence. And remember, women are on the beauty industry payroll too, do not trust them when it comes to advice on what constitutes being beautiful.

My advice to any woman is that she should feel comfortable in who she is and make her own standards of beauty. If you want to wear something to look or feel beautiful, do it for yourself, though there is no problem in wearing something that your partner finds attractive, but he should also do the same for you. This is all part of maintaining a healthy partnership. Above everything else you should know that you are beautiful and need no one's approval or acceptance.

I hope that whilst reading this you do not think that I am pitting men against women; I am merely showing how the two are under pressure to look a certain way based on the ideas of a few men and women in the beauty industry. These ideas of beauty are driven by Capitalism and corporate profits for their shareholders. All men are not the bad guys here, most guys do not tell women how to dress, in fact I would say it is women telling other women how to dress. Women need to stop projecting their insecurities onto other women, they need to support one another to dress and look the way they want and not how fashion dictates. They need to help end bullying and 'body shaming'.

I have spoken to enough women to realise that the Capitalist based beauty industry is telling women that they have certain physical flaws, and exploits them in order to make a quick buck and ideally a lifelong customer. Men and women need to search for inner beauty and remove these superficial ideas of what constitutes beauty. Once they are at peace with their appearance, no amount of manipulative advertising will affect them. One day we will all see through the nonsense in such adverts telling us 'You can have long and luscious lashes all day long' or 'You are so worth it'.

It is time to embrace humans in all their natural beauty, colour and diverse shapes.

<u>Talking To Myself?</u>

So, before I begin to write, Facebook asks me "What's on your mind?" This is a question we (humanity) need to ask one another more often. I believe that worrying and keeping things to oneself seems to be the way for many people, especially men.

The sad reality is that keeping it all inside eats away at us, killing our very being. In Japan (and in many other Asian countries) many men commit suicide due to their problems, society deeming it culturally unacceptable for men to speak about their worries. Even here in England, and no doubt in many other parts of Europe too, men resort to this 'way out'. It is *apparently* better to fall on your own sword - to *honour* oneself and family. This is *not* the solution however. Men and women have the same emotions and need to talk about their problems. If we close ourselves off or put up an emotional wall we'll all suffer. We need to talk, to let out the deep-seated fears within us.

This is a tough and unforgiving economic world where money is seen as the *be all* and *end all* of our problems. We lose our minds (literally in some cases) making profits for corporations that hide their wealth in offshore accounts while our own families, communities and people are left neglected or starved of funding. We are not machines or just their 'human resources'. We are human beings, flesh, bone, and with complex emotions. We need our communities and need one another. No one is an island.

We can remedy this situation however, by talking more and spending little or no time worrying, which will help if we are having emotional or financial problems. We can set up our own local credit unions, and not be at the mercy of banks and interest lending that leaves many people homeless. There is a lot of support out there for anyone who needs help. We just need to learn how to talk more openly and support one another.

The ideology of 'Individualism' is killing our communities. It is creating more people with mental health problems, more lonely pensioners, more single parents, more feral children and more crime. Every creature lives in a community, from birds, insects to humans. We are not meant to be solitary creatures stuck in a show kitchen in a show house. What is the point of being independent when no one comes to visit you? What is so good about being a lonely old man or woman? We need each other to thrive, to keep our communities and us alive.

Are We All ET? (Extra Terrestrial)

God, the universe, evolution or nature, whatever or whomever you believe created you; one thing is for certain, that you were created for a purpose. The force that created you felt it important that you play a pivotal role in this world. You may not comprehend your reason for being here, question your existence, or even feel like you belong, but you should have the conviction that you matter.

We are all made up of the same elements. We have four blood types among our species. We are one race of people and come in various shades, shapes and sizes. It is no coincidence that the universe and all that is created within it is made up of the same 96 elements that we find here on earth. Our DNA is unique to each of us, our fingerprints too. We are all unique, one off originals, never to be repeated. This is proof for me that the force that created us has a purpose for us. Think of your DNA and fingerprints as your identity card, passport or driver's license, they are unique to you and will never be reissued to anyone else. Everything about our body points to the fact that we are unique. Our very matter - matters.

We can agree or disagree about who or what created us, and about what our purpose in life really is, but we cannot disagree that a 'force' created us for a reason. The force of God, nature, evolution or intelligent design made a decision to create us in the shape and form that we are in today. That 'force' chose the shape of our planet, trees, clouds and the very universe we occupy. That force, we can agree, is a super intelligent one, and one that we will never be able to fully comprehend in our lifetime.

We were brought into existence because it was important for us to think, to observe and contemplate our very being. Unlike animals, humans were given the ability to think about their existence, to create many languages and forms of communication, such as the Internet, film, Art and literature. Why have we been singled out for these creative forms of communication? Why do the many electrical devices, forms of media, and transportation now bind us across the world?

We are unlike any other species on Earth. We suffer from illness, aches and pains; we depend on our teachers and doctors to help get us through this life. We are dependent on so many things and can never be as independent as say a polar bear or wolf. Why did we need the comfort of a fire to keep us warm and to cook our food? Again this is another sign of our being very different to other creatures with which we share this amazing planet.

My personal belief is that we are not of this earth, and that our origins are from another realm, we are all extra-terrestrials. I do not mean this in a 'green aliens from Mars' kind of way, or that we are literally 'alien' in our origin, but that we had a previous home, and are destined for that home again after we leave this world.

The gravity of the earth does not suit us, hence the backaches and sore limbs we succumb to. We get sunburnt if we stay out in the sun for too long. If evolution has evolved us to the top of the species ladder, why do we suffer from these ailments? Surely we should have evolved much stronger backs and a tougher skin?

As I said earlier in this blog, we can agree to disagree but these points are worth thinking over. Keep an open mind.

Had We Two Hearts

'Had we two hearts and one were heartbroken, the second would allow us continue living.'

This is an interesting thought, but something we might not ever ponder over. We have only one heart however, and that is why we must be careful not to break it, or more importantly, break someone else's.

The heart literally 'thinks' independently, has its own 'intelligence' and can make up its own 'mind'. We often hear of some poor soul suffering from brain damage, but there is also such a thing as 'heart damage'. The damage to the heart, just like any done to the brain, is difficult to repair, and often lasts a very long time, or even a lifetime. People often die of a broken heart.

Why am I saying all of this? Well, I see so many people breaking hearts and being heartbroken that I am beginning to wonder if they even care anymore. I see many acting as though we all have a spare heart, as though we can just get over any heartbreak and any hurt thrown at us. Once damaged, the heart will self-repair, but at what cost and over how much time?

There is a lot of research showing the detrimental effects, especially upon women, from relationships that have ended badly. An individual can be left deeply wounded and emotionally scarred for life. Over many years and many relationships the heart becomes numb; it no longer feels anything or trusts anyone. People lose their confidence and begin to experience depression, become isolated, and we know many of those heartbroken sadly go on to self-harm. Some will commit suicide or a crime of passion. How many times have you heard of boyfriends or ex-husbands killing their former partner? How many people with broken hearts have committed suicide? We need to help end such crimes and tragedies.

Before you give your heart to someone, just ask yourself, will they treasure and care for it as though it were their own? Will they care for it as you wish? If the answer is no to these questions, do not proceed any further. There are already too many broken hearts in the world; and those doing the breaking care not for one more being thrown onto the heart scrap heap.

We only have one heart; we need to take care of it, as well as the hearts of others.

It is better to remain single than to give your heart to a monster.

The Madness of Meat

'Cows and chickens are being injected with hormones, steroids, and God only knows what else!'

In 1993, the Food and Drug Administration (FDA) approved recombinant bovine growth hormone (rBGH), a synthetic cow hormone that spurs milk production when injected into dairy cows. These cows may even be advertised as being 'free range'. Personally I'd say such cows are anything but "free". They are experiments, beasts of burden, and an unholy creation. The poor creatures can barely stand, yet their skeleton is expected to adjust to their new weight gain. It's an abomination of nature, or rather man, as we are going against nature by creating such creatures.

Imagine what the side affect will be after years of consuming such 'modified' animals? Actually, you won't be able to, as there is no data at present. This reminds me of the 'Mad Cow Disease' we had back in the 1990s, when cows were being force fed ground up meat in the form of pellets. That's right; herbivores (plant eaters) were being forced into becoming omnivores (plant and meat eaters). That was a recipe for disaster. Going against thousands of years of nature will never produce anything good in the long term. The meat industry will make a tidy profit however, kill millions in the process, and no doubt give others a host of illnesses, but the gain will only ever be short term.

We are partly responsible for the cruelty inflicted upon these creatures. The meat and dairy industry supplies our demand for meat and dairy products. Whether it's steak, ice-cream or cheese on our pizzas, it's these poor cows and other creatures that have to pay the price. The food industry is making us into an obese generation. Gluttony is becoming the norm. Being overweight is no longer seen as unhealthy. When people say they are of "average" build they actually mean 'overweight'. If you're slim to athletic people call you "skinny". I can't help but think that doctors and our media are telling us to consume more in order to make us unhealthy and thus help sell more food and drugs. I mean do we really need to be consuming 2400 calories per day? I personally don't think so. Our bodies are designed to operate on far less, as they are extremely economical. We should be fasting more not eating more.

So many animals are being 'pumped up' to feed our insatiable appetites. Chickens arc injected with chemicals, as are sheep, lamb and even fish. Soon there will be no more 'organic' or 'free range' animals left, as the pressure to supply more for less will increase in what is already a tough food market. We know that chicken meat for example is really cheap, but it is injected with water to make it seem heavier than it really is. Just fry some chicken breast and see how much water comes out and how the meat shrinks. Remember the beef that wasn't really beef? It was mixed with horsemeat. You may recall the horsemeat scandal a few years back. Dead horses were being cut up and mixed with beef coming from Poland and Romania. No one knows where the meat originated. It was found out to be widespread across European butchers and supermarkets. No one was prosecuted to my knowledge. What else is being mixed into our meat? Dog meat? Rat meat? Donkey meat?

For thousands of years humanity has been consuming meat, but not at the rate we are consuming it today. Meat used to be a luxury, once the food of kings. Our bodies are adapted to live on a 20/80 ratio of meat and vegetables. Vegetables should be our main food intake, and meat shouldn't be consumed more than once a week. Meat can be taken out of our diet altogether, as any vegan will tell you. I think of myself as part vegetarian. I have meat maybe once a week, and rarely if ever eat meat from take-outs or restaurants. There are too many people out there faking turkey for lamb, or horsemeat for beef. I just don't have any confidence in the food industry. I will have soya milk to cut down on my milk intake. I also make sure the milk is sourced from a farm that doesn't use steroids or hormones on their cows. If you live near a farm you should inquire as to how they raise their animals.

If we look at meat consumption from a world religion point of view, we will find that meat is rarely and often never consumed (according to scripture and religious tradition). In Buddhism a vegetarian diet is encouraged, Hindus prefer a vegetarian diet to minimize the suffering of animals, in Sikhism a lacto-vegetarian diet is served in the gurdwara, and encouraged in everyday life, in Islam meat was rarely eaten by the Prophet Muhammad, and if it was, it was rarely if ever on the bone, and in small cube pieces, maybe eaten once a month. This is the same pattern in Christianity and Judaism. The religious leaders of the world's religions ate very little if any meat. It is only since the rise of the consumer society, fast food and the 'eat-out' and 'foodie' culture that meat has been consumed in such large amounts.

We know that 95% of health ailments are linked to diet. I believe that our consumption of meat is literally decreasing our life span. It is no coincidence that diabetes, high blood pressure and cardiovascular problems are on the rise. The number of people suffering from heart burn, chest pains, strokes and poor eyesight is worrying, especially when it's occurring in those below the age of 40.

I'll tell you a little known secret about another animal that suffers for 'fast food' demands, the pig. If the pig weren't slaughtered, it would soon die of a heart attack. That's how unhealthy it is before it's served to you on a plate. Pork consumption is linked to seventy diseases. Let that sink in.

You may want to change your diet for the sake of your own health, and more importantly, the suffering of animals. The less meat we eat, the less they have to suffer. I hope we can reverse this steroid meat trend and go back to real 'organic' farming.

<u>You Are Already Complete</u>

I am sure many of you will have heard people say things like 'He makes me feel complete' or 'My life is complete with her', etc. These statements might seem harmless enough, a mere gesture of love and appreciation; only if we were to think deeper on such statements we would see that there is a fundamental flaw here. They point to a lack of confidence.

You see, we come into this world already 'complete', but for some reason or other, we are told that we "need someone" to make life, and us, 'complete'. Why does society perpetuate this idea? Are we not already complete as an individual? I often hear people say things like "She is thirty now, she should get married" or "You are thirty-five now, you should own your own house". What nonsense is this?

Living a complete life requires self-confidence and self-belief. If we believe from an early age that we are complete, we will not need to think of ourselves as being incomplete or insufficient. We should not feel 'needy' or 'lacking' in any respect. We will end up making the wrong decisions if we do not believe in our own abilities. We need to tackle those people that will use us or make us feel inferior. Needy people take from us making us feel incomplete, and when this happens over time it can leave a big void in our own lives. People that give and never receive often end up lonely and full of regrets. Giving is good, but we should not allow people to take, take, take, it must be a reciprocal relationship. We live in an age of the 'freeloader' and career 'benefit scrounger'. Be careful whom you choose as friends and acquaintances.

I hope that you all feel 'complete' as an individual, and that you grow stronger in your own abilities each and every day. Stay strong and secure within yourself.

<u>Meditation and Mindfulness</u>

This could be one of my longest posts but I will try to keep it short. I began meditating on a daily basis some three years ago, nothing too time consuming or deep, just ten minutes per day, and occasionally in the evening. There is a lot of evidence to suggest that meditation makes you healthier and happier. I would like to think that this is true about myself. It is of course impossible to be perpetually 'happy', but we can have happy moments, and be content for the best part of our lives.

Meditation is used as a therapy to prevent depression, stress and other cognitive ailments too. It benefits the brain in so many ways. I wish doctors would prescribe meditation to depressed patients instead of medication.

No, you will not need to sit under a tree assuming the position of the Buddha, though that would do you no harm. Long-term meditation reduces loss of memory and increases brain volume, thus allowing your brain a longer and more active lifespan; no wonder sages and prophets over the centuries have used meditation in their daily lives. Meditation is like coffee, as it energises the mind and body, only it is a much healthier boost (too much coffee keeps your brain over energised and can lead to stress). Meditation is also a better alternative to medicine. It is also a great immune system booster. Meditating for just twenty minutes is equivalent to ninety minutes of sleep, so it is great for power breaks on long drives, or during a work break if you are feeling lethargic (don't touch that coffee!). Employers really should invest in 'quiet rooms' for their employees.

I won't go into too much detail on meditation, but I will give you some basic information to hopefully get you interested. There are ten stages of meditation, or 'levels'. Each of these levels will help you improve your meditative skills. By practicing you will master a certain level, at which you can remain or move on. As you are unique you will find a stage that suits you best. You do not have to compete with other people, as their needs are very different to your own. It's all about your own attitude and what you wish to gain from meditating. There is no competitiveness involved. You are free to meditate at your leisure.

There are no short cuts to meditation, it takes time and dedication on your part, but it is very achievable and worthwhile. Do not worry if you make progress one week only to slip back the next. This is perfectly natural. After many years of meditating I still have good or not so good meditation sessions. It all depends on what is going on in my life. Some people think it can take many years to achieve a good meditative state, this is not true however, as I experienced some of my most spiritual states very early on, and within only a few weeks of practicing. Meditation is not a linear process, you will move between various stages. In time you will find a good mental 'place' that works best for you. The secret is not time, it's effort and perseverance. You really can do it.

The type of meditation I do personally is called 'mindfulness'; it is a 'waking state' in which you focus on the now, forgetting about the past and not thinking about the future. Monks use this type of meditation to live in the present moment (note: I am against a life of celibacy as it is unnatural to the human race). Try meditating at around dawn, before you go to work or later in the evening after you come home. Find a comfortable place, in a comfortable environment, and sit cross-legged on a cushion or blanket. Close your eyes and think of a word to make you forget about everything. I use words such as 'empty' or 'now' but yours could be any word, as long as it brings about a mind 'clearing' or 'reset'. You may have to try several words depending on how you feel. I find that thinking of happy memories helps brings about a state of calm.

You might feel silly at first but just wait until you see the benefits, you will soon be meditating daily. If you search online for 'meditation' you will find many books and articles to help you improve your technique. I found several good books in my local library. You can search for classes in your locality too.

I wish you all the best in your quest for physical peace and contentment of mind.

<u>Debt - The Real WMD</u>
(Weapon of Mass Destruction)

"I am free!"

How many of you can say this? I know that I am really 'free' because I have no debt. I stayed clear of credit cards, loans and mortgages. I know many have no choice, but most of us do. I say this because I always hear people tell me that it is better to buy a house on a mortgage than to rent. The same people tell me years later that they are in debt, that they are struggling to make payments and that they cannot afford to go on holiday, let alone relocate to a different area or move abroad. Many are in negative equity on the house they paid too much for, and now that same property is worth half of its original value due to an economic decline and the area lacking development. I know people with mortgages (mortgage means 'death pledge' in French) of £120,000 to £200,000, they will have to pay back £240,000 to £400,000 in thirty to forty years. Why? Surely this is financial entrapment?

Homes are made of wood, bricks and cement; they are not really worth so much money. An average house price in London is £500,000, and in the North it is around £300,000. Who on this planet can afford such prices? Londoners are being priced out of their own city, and their city will soon be the exclusive resort of the super rich, what with the Russians, Chinese and Arab developers buying out huge chunks of land for development, as well as buying up million pound properties in the city.

House prices in England were once affordable. In the 1970s a three-bedroom house in the north of England could be bought for as little as £3000, the same house now will cost between £125,000 to £240,000. In Manchester it is around £300,000 to £600,000. The reason for this price increase is due to private banks playing with the rate of interest and inflation also raising prices. Mortgage lenders are also to blame, artificially hiking up house valuation prices in order to gain a greater piece of the commission. Two potential buyers, who do not have even a tenth of the value of a desired property, will bid with one another backed by their lender. One bids at £100,000 and the other bids £110,000, this continues until the two foolish bidders reach a figure of around £200,000, for a property whose actual value is no more than £30,000 in real terms of physical property. The bank wins every time, leaving the homeowner to pay off double over the next thirty years. See how quickly house prices will come down if we refuse to take out their rotten mortgages and loans. We will soon see 'real' prices return. We can then afford to buy a house in cash.

Of course governments are in on the act too, refusing to build enough social housing in order to drive those desperate folks to the home loan providers. Private landlords are not regulated either, their monthly rents can be almost the same as a monthly mortgage or loan payment. I would still sooner rent however, not wanting to be enslaved or suffer the mental anguish of a lifetime of debt. We need to put pressure on the Government to build more social housing, as there are currently over two million people on the council (social housing) waiting list. Homes can be built for less than £60,000 so there is no excuse for not spending our taxes on affordable housing. The world governments have for far too long served the interests of corporations and banks. The private banks caused the financial crisis yet we taxpayers have had to bail them out to the tune of £4 billion! That is just in the UK. It is a disgrace and frankly criminal. The Government could have built homes with the bailout money or set up local cooperative community banks and credit unions.

I recently met a teacher who is in the final year of her mortgage, she is now aged fifty-nine, a year from retirement, and she is alone, making the last payments herself, her divorce and partner leaving her with the mortgage did not help. She told me that taking out a mortgage was the worst decision she had ever made, thinking at the time that they could both pay it off in fifteen years, and could leave the family house to their children. Their children have moved out, got their own rented properties or are working abroad. Did they even want the house? It's unlikely. Money problems are also a major factor in a couple's marriage breaking up. Mortgages end many marriages.

Debt is the anchor that keeps the ship in harbour; it is a noose around the neck as we balance on the chair of life, and the tightrope we must walk, never knowing when we might fall. The banks are glorified casinos, and just as with the casino, the house always wins.

Look at how the current economic crisis occurred and you will soon realize that it was all the fault of the banks, lending money they did not have, only one real dollar or pound backs up every ten they lend out. The whole system is corrupt, and it has brought Europe to its knees, and even America has not escaped its rot. The U.S. is in $23 trillion of debt (as of 2017), and has now been downgraded to AA status; down from its previous AAA status, meaning its ability to pay back loans is in doubt. The United Kingdom is in £1.7 trillion of debt (as of 2017), but to whom? The International Monetary Fund, that's who, a private bank, just like the Federal

Reserve and Bank of England. Banks are the new slave masters, destroying lives and nations overnight.

I recently read an article about the amount of student debt in the U.S. causing many girls to work in strip clubs or even prostitution; many do this work to pay initial college fees that are around $20,000 per year. This situation is being repeated in Greece, just do an online search and you will find many stories by credible journalists from broadsheet news sources. Greece has never been so poor; it is likened to a third world nation. Interest Banking has ruined Europe, and it is the main cause of Africa's poverty and continuing lack of development. Nations are put into so much debt that they are literally taken over, even taken hostage by the banks. Interest banking also creates crime, poverty and war.

Interest Banking is causing a mass social crisis and mass exodus. It is preventing couples from getting a place of their own, some graduates have even moved back in with their parents, as they simply cannot afford to live alone. Why can't someone earning £20,000 to £30,000 each year no longer afford their own house? Even with our degrees we cannot get onto the property ladder, as most of us have student loan debts of around £27,000 to pay off. I was fortunate enough to qualify for a student grant. I studied part time over six years, alongside my part time job.

I know of couples looking to buy reasonable properties, nothing fancy, not in a great area, but the prices begin at £200,000, so they would have to find a £20,000 deposit before even trying to purchase, then there is those "better" properties starting at £300,000. I mean who on earth wants £600,000 of debt over forty years? There is also the 'Early Repayment Fee', so if you are able to pay off your loan early the bank will charge you a fee! Am I the only one getting mad here? These people are legal criminals.

The 'banksters' are not interested in clearing your debt, they want you enslaved from cradle to grave, with their worthless paper money that they print whenever they feel like it! 'Quantitative Easing' is the fancy term they use, or basically printing new money. They say money does not grow on trees, this is true, but it does grow in banks, out of cyber air!

My advice to you all is to remain debt free, to not be enslaved. Buy a home abroad if you wish, they are much cheaper than in the United Kingdom for sure. Try a different part of the country, or simply rent. If we do not help end this cycle of debt we will all soon be homeless. Just look at how many homeless we have already, how many families are being thrown out by bailiffs? Some of the landlords are in the same dilemma, buying homes on interest mortgages, and then passing on those debts to their tenants. A below average two bedroom flat in the North of England goes for about £600 per month, add that to the £120 council tax, plus bills, food, etc. and you are looking at around £900 per month before you have even spent anything on yourself or your family! You will also want to think about whether you can afford to run a car with all of this to pay. This is the age of debt, and only the smart will stay afloat.

Let me also just mention the new craze of 'Crypto Currency'. Onecoin has recently shut down its operations and is under investigation (as of February 2018). Many people have lost tens of thousands overnight. I know of one lady who lost £35,000. The crypto currency creators use a pyramid system to earn money out of desperate people that are looking for a quick investment, or 'get rich quick' scheme. These moneymaking schemes were big in the 1990s too.

It amazes me that so many people still fall for such pyramid schemes. I think it's easy to trick people out of their money nowadays; they don't want to work hard but do want to get rich overnight. Greed usually ends in debt, but hard work brings success.

Stay free, stay smart, and avoid debt.

<u>Dreams of My Own</u>

We are all familiar with the idea of 'pushy parents' or 'competitive parents'. This is part of the cultural make up in most societies, though it varies in degree. It is very common in Asian communities, for example an Asian parent who happens to be a doctor will want his son or daughter to also become a doctor. If one of the parents is an engineer or pharmacist they will want their children to follow in these professions too. There is a lot of pressure on children to fulfil the dreams of their parents. Often the parents are from poor and uneducated backgrounds; they may never have realized their own dreams and ambitions and wish to live out their dreams through their children.

In Western culture we also see this 'living out' of parents' dreams in children. A father will often say 'That's my boy' or 'That's daddy's girl', etc. There is a particular pride in children following their parents' dreams and doing well. This can be very difficult for children to maintain however, as they more often than not will have their own dreams and ambitions.

I have met many unfulfilled young men and women that are working in their parents' business, or have followed the same profession, whether engineering or medicine, etc. When I have asked them if this is what they dreamed of doing after graduating, many reply saying that their parents wanted them to become a doctor or engineer, etc. I have met many people with university degrees who work in fast food or retail, who never intended to, but who were coerced into the family business, feeling a sense of familial duty.

I am not sure if parents still ask their children what they would like to become, or if they support them in their dreams. I know they support them academically and financially, but I cannot help but feel that many parents coerce their children, and mould them into what they as parents want them to become. I think this is why many people in their late thirties and early forties become disillusioned with their careers, as it was not their first love or passion, they instead followed the advice of their parents or peers and chose the "safe" option. The 'job for life' however no longer applies. People want to try various occupations.

I have seen the extreme and abusive side of parenting too. Some parents will disown their children if they do not follow the family tradition of working in the family business. If they choose another career other than that which their parents desire, they can be abused emotionally and physically. Some parents will even stop supporting them financially. Their siblings, or extended family will often ostracize them too. This level of abuse is more prevalent than we think. It is more common towards girls than boys, especially within Asian communities.

In Chinese communities there is also a lot of pressure put upon boys - often an only child. This will be in part due to the 'One Child' policy in China. Girls tend to be allowed to study any subject, as they will marry and go to another home, whereas the boys will stay and support their parents. I can appreciate that often a family business is the only viable option for work and an income, but other possibilities should not be ruled out, as a child may have an alternative or new business idea. The parents should at least consider such ideas. It may actually be more successful and more profitable than the current family business.

I think parents need to have more faith and trust in their children's abilities. Children will become successful in whatever they choose to do, as their passion and ambition will motivate them, as well as the support they receive from their families.

I do not want to meet any more adults in unhappy professions. Support your children with *their* dreams, and not your own.

<u>Is Money Your God?</u>

'The economy goes up, and we smile, the economy goes down, and we cry.'

Have we been reduced to slaves that worship the economy gods? Have our lives and happiness become so dependent upon this money-monster that we now live in constant fear? It would seem so. We anxiously wait for the banks to lower interest rates, for our leaders to give us good news of economic growth and job security. We live in a state of constant insecurity, and are perpetually at the mercy of banks. What kind of existence is this? We need to end this daily trauma.

There is no 'Work and life balance'. This is merely an empty slogan just like 'You only live once' or 'Support the troops'. We can see around us the damage caused by our dependence on financial institutions, or rather financial 'instability'. Entire economies crash in a day of trading and people are left bankrupt overnight, whether it is in Libya, Venezuela or Greece. Businesses go bankrupt within minutes and workers are laid off with little notice. This is the harshness of our so-called "progressive" and "democratic" Capitalism. It is a system that benefits the few and robs the many.

The economic demi-gods throw us scraps that fall from the moneylenders' table. If the economy is strong we are rewarded, if it is not we are given nothing, and austerity measures are put into place. Even the scraps are soon stopped.

"FEED ME BY SPENDING WHAT LITTLE MONEY YOU HAVE!" the economic gods demand. "SPEND! SPEND! SPEND!" They cry. "FEED ME!" And of course we do. We feed the economic gods with our money, spending what little we have on clothes and gadgets that we do not even need. If we do not have any money we just buy expensive goods on credit cards or take out loans. We must spend, right? We have to feed the economic gods or they will threaten us with poverty. What a tragic existence.

Have we really become reduced to trembling slaves? Are we really so weak that we live in constant fear of threats of poverty by a handful of banks? They are certainly very good at keeping us in a state of fear and in need. If you take one thing from this article, take this; that the banks want to trap you into debt and they want you trapped for life. No bank wants to "help" you pay off your debt. They want a customer (consumer/slave) for life. It is even better for them if you leave your loan or mortgage to your children. They can then enslave them for life too.

You only have to read the many articles online or in your local newspaper to see how many people commit suicide because they have no money, have lost their homes, or have been made redundant. Are these people making the ultimate 'human' sacrifice to their economic gods? In India for example, eighty percent of farmers commit suicide due to being unable to pay off bank debts (source: Indianexpress.com). The evil institutions they call "banks", are in my opinion, deliberately trapping the largely uneducated and poor into a cycle of debt. The 1% thrives whilst 99% die.

Debt and austerity measures are significant factors in the rising number of suicides of young men in the United Kingdom. Between 2008 and 2010 there were 30 - 40 thousand suicide attempts due to the economic downturn (source: Oxford University). I am appalled by these figures. Having no money is *not* a reason to take your own life. We are human beings and our lives are of great value, even sacred. Debt related suicides have also soared across much of Europe due to the economic collapse in nations such as Greece, Ireland and Portugal. The Interest Banking System is literally killing people on a genocidal scale. Add to this the student debt that is also claiming more lives than ever before.

Many female students now work as prostitutes to cover their rent and student fees or to pay off loans. Interest and debt are nothing less than weapons of mass destruction. They are the destroyer of worlds.

Is an individual's worth linked to their bank account? Does money really make the man? Are the poor a burden and the rich our royalty? This is not what life is about. We are not here to accumulate paper money, gold or silver. Our purpose in life is not for hoarding billions of dollars and declaring our wealth to the world. I see this illness spreading to the poorest regions of the world, where huge infrastructures are being built adjacent to slums, where billionaires live side by side with the most poor that make up the majority in that nation.

How much money do we need to live our sixty or seventy years on earth? Even if we live to be a hundred we could never be in need of a billion dollars, or even a million for that matter. This greed for money is a mental health problem; it is a sickness of the heart and mind. It needs to be cured.

I am not saying don't be successful, and not to make a lot of money, I am saying don't let it consume you, or make you greedy. I would love to make lots of money so I could set up a charity, or donate more to charities. Money in of itself is not bad; it's what you do with it that matters. Hoarding it benefits no one. Offshore accounts starve nations of their wealth.

It is time to stop worshiping the economic demi-gods and start serving humanity once more. We need to look after one another, not other peoples' bank accounts.

We are not here to please shareholders and corporations. It is time for change. We need to say no to loans and mortgages, we must keep away from buying on credit and buy only what we can afford, and not what we want. It is time for us to think about our own well-being, not what others will think of us. It does not matter if you drive an old car, if you have a low salary or if you did not go to college. What really matters is your life and those near and dear to you.

Stay debt free and you will not be a slave to money.

<u>What Is Love?</u>

This week has brought me into contact with many people that have asked me about Love. I have also read many, many comments on social media regarding Love and how to define it. When we think of Love we imagine it being between a couple, parents and children, and even pets and their owners. But what is Love? Are there different *types* of love?

Love is Love, it asks and wants for nothing. It is pure. Can you think of a time when you fell in love or felt love? Can you recall that pure, unadulterated and honest feeling? Remember the elation and how Love pushed out all prejudices and demands?

Once Love begins to ask and demand of others it is no longer Love, but rather a 'conditional' love, a 'contractual' love. If this is what your idea of Love is then you need to mature as an individual and find out more about life and how Love works. The nature of Love is something that requires knowledge and understanding, as well as feeling. Love is such a powerful emotion that it can create great things but also destroy them. It is an emotion that must be tamed, just like anger. Do not let Love overpower you, be moderate in all your feelings.

How often do we hear people say; 'Do this for me and I will love you', 'Do that for me and I will love you more' or 'If you don't do it I won't will love any more.' This playing with Love and diluting it is wrong. Do not take what is pure and make it something inferior. No one wants diluted milk or honey. If someone is offering Love then they should not cheat the person by giving him or her a diluted form of it. If there are to be conditions to such 'love' they ought to be stated in advance, so that a person may make an informed decision on whether to accept or reject it. The same goes for diluted milk and honey.

I feel that a lot of problems in this world have come about due the absence of real Love and the presence of a lesser 'love'.

We really need to be more honest with each other. Don't promise what you won't deliver.

The Emotional Orphan

What is an 'emotional orphan'? Well, I can say I have known a few, and met many more. I recall the first being a young boy of twelve. His father was in the British Army, his mother worked full time as a nurse. He had one older sister but they were worlds apart. This boy had everything in the material sense, a great house, fashionable clothes and the best toys. What he did not have however, was time with his parents. His father had spent most of his time away from home, and his mother worked long and unsociable hours in a very stressful profession. He pretty much raised himself.

The second emotional orphan was a boy I met at junior high school. His father was a pilot and his mother was an airhostess. You can imagine how little contact he had with *his* parents. He was also an only child. I think being an only child must be so difficult, and coming from a family of five siblings I know I would have *really* struggled with life had *I* been alone.

The boy I knew had lots of money given to him, all the toys and clothes he wanted, new bikes and trainers, etc. but little or no time with his parents. He would spend most of his time with his grandparents. I often wonder why couples have a child or children, I mean if they have not got any time for them. We now live in a time of broken families and lost children.

The third emotional orphan was a young girl that I worked with at a local primary school. Her father was working six days a week and never had any time for her. I guess I became a kind of surrogate father figure to her. She would talk to me about her day, what she got up to at the weekend, her hobbies and interests. I felt sad that this girl's father was missing out on the best years of her life. Her mother did not understand her, as she had come from abroad and the difference in culture and language was somewhat of a barrier. They could not have been more different.

The fourth emotional orphan was a young boy I had also worked with at a local primary school. It was all angst with him however. I felt he was taking out his angry feelings on me to compensate for his absent father. For an eight-year-old boy from a nice family he had so much anger and social issues to deal with. Again it was clear to me that he just needed a father figure in his life. His own father was too busy with work and rarely if ever came to pick him up from school. I managed to impart *some* parental control and eventually formed a good understanding with the boy.

There is a pattern of anti-social behaviour in children who have little emotional contact with their parents. These 'emotional orphans' go on to have emotional problems as adults and find it hard to bond with their own future partners and children.

So, going back to my original question. What is an emotional orphan? Emotional orphans are those children that have parents, siblings, aunties and uncles, cousins, etc. only with little emotional contact with any of these relatives. Often they will have some bond with their grandparents, at least until their early teens. Grandparents sadly do not live for very long. Both of my grandparents passed away in their 70s.

The emotional orphan has plenty of toys and nice clothes, money to spend on fine things, but nothing in terms of rewarding relationships. Often they are an only child, or one of two siblings, the other sibling is usually the opposite gender. The parents will not have much if any time for this emotional orphan, as they are too busy with their careers. The orphan looks "happy" to those around him or her, there is no need to feel any immediate concern for their physical safety, however they are as lonely as any orphan in care.

These emotional orphans have few friends, and those they do have will move on in life, that is how friendships come and go. They may find some stable friends in their teens or early twenties, but they usually lack the skills or confidence to form consistent and meaningful relationships. This is more of a problem nowadays with fickle friendships being made and broken online. Online bullying is rampant too.

The emotional orphan never really bonds with his parents; he or she often feels alone. The bonding process of parent and child is something we know to be of great importance in the animal kingdom let alone the human one. If this 'bonding' and close emotional attachment is not done in the first few years of a child's life it can have a huge impact on their psychological well-being and later adult life.

So next time you speak to or work with a child, do not assume that they are emotionally well, that they are happy in life. It is always worth finding out about a child's emotional well being, as well as their outward physical and material appearance. As a former educator I was taught to recognize the signs of emotional trauma, signs that told me 'all was not well'.

As parents we must do all we can to provide our children with emotional as well as material security. Their emotional needs are just as important if not more important than their physical needs. Parents need to spend time with their children, not money.

I hope you make a difference in your children's lives.

<u>Summer Love</u>

I was 'googling' the other day and came across a post on Google's home page. I took a screenshot of it as a reminder. The part that stood out for me was:

"Watching the sunrise outdoors statistically increases your odds of having a good day."

I have long held a fascination of the sun, the moon, and astronomy in general. I have enjoyed taking pictures of sunsets and sunrises for many years now, as I am sure many of you will have too. I always get up before sunrise, this is firstly to meditate, and secondly to enjoy and capture the birth of a new day. After all these years I am still in awe of each sunrise, and can honestly say, at least for myself, that it really does give *me* a good day *and* a good feeling.

There is something primal in witnessing a sunrise, it awakens something in the subconscious mind, releasing chemicals in the brain that energise the body. I don't know if there is a scientific explanation, but I do know that it benefits me.

So no matter where you are in the world, I encourage you witness this heavenly spectacle regularly, it far outshines (pun intended) any form of "entertainment" your television can provide. I encourage you all to connect with this daily natural phenomenon to see if you have better days too. You will feel energized from the moment you see the sun breaking over the horizon.

WARNING: I know this might seem obvious, but never look directly at the sun, even with a camera, telescope sun-filter or binoculars. I have read many cases of people suffering eye damage, especially children; even sunglasses do not fully protect your eyes from harm. Don't take the risk.

<u>Repetitive Separation Syndrome</u>

Children are suffering from repetitive separation from parents and extended relatives on a worrying scale. I see it leading to more mental health problems.

I have coined the term Repetitive Separation (RSS) Syndrome myself, as I could not find any term that defines repetitive separation. I will mention the symptoms which I believe are indicators for the condition, however, I am not a medical practitioner or psychologist, I am merely providing you with my observations as an educator with experience of working with young children for nearly ten years.

I first noticed the symptoms of repetitive separation syndrome whilst working at a local primary school. I spent a considerable amount of time working in the school nursery, where I would teach small groups of children aged between three and four years of age. It was at the beginning of the new school year that I would notice children experiencing the worst of separation. The children's parents would drop them off and spend ten to fifteen minutes observing them from a distance. The class teacher would request that each parent leave once his or her child had begun to settle down. Of course a child would eventually notice that their parent had disappeared. This is when the 'trauma' would begin.

You might think that *trauma* is too strong a term, but let me ask you this, what if you were out with your child and you suddenly noticed that they were missing? Would that be a *traumatic* experience? Would you panic or scream? I imagine every parent would. So what about your child? You see, parents 'sneak away' when toys or other children distract their three year old. When a child needs to see their parent later, they are nowhere to be found. Now imagine this on a daily basis, over several weeks? Pretty cruel don't you think?

I can recall one particular child crying for a whole two months. Every day he would be dropped off, and every day the parent would disappear once the child was distracted. The poor child would then cry for hours. I recall one day when things got so bad that they had to call his mother to come and pick him up early. Personally I see this daily routine as child abuse, and yes, this *is* another strong term, but I feel it *is* justified. Imagine if someone took their dog for a walk; let it off the leash to run in the park, and then left? What would happen to the dog? Would you view the dog owner as being cruel? I *certainly* would.

I do not know at what age children start nursery or kindergarten in the East, but in the West, most schools will accept a child at the age of two to three years of age. In many European countries, such as Finland and Norway, children start school at the age of seven. This makes much more sense than having them start at three. It is all fun and games at age three anyhow, nothing academic or essential.

The constant trauma of being separated can cut the emotional attachment to a parent; and have a detrimental impact on a child's wellbeing in later adult life. It can cause Separation Anxiety Disorder (SAD), which is the excessive or inappropriate anxiety of being separated from parents or the home, often beginning before the age of eighteen. Reactive Attachment Disorder is another risk (RAD); this is when the child becomes excessively inhibited, hyper-vigilant, ambivalent, and experiences social interaction problems.

The study of separation is a relatively new science, although much has been learned in this area. We know for example that the following symptoms are attributed to repetitive separation over a period of months or years: 'recurrent and excessive distress about being away from home or parents, constant excessive worry about losing a parent to an illness or a disaster, constant worry that something bad will happen, such as being lost or kidnapped, irrational fear of separation from parents, refusing to be away from home because of fear of separation, not wanting to be alone and without a parent in the house, repeated nightmares about separation, frequent complaints of headaches, stomach-aches or other symptoms when separation from a parent is anticipated. (Source: Amy Bruce, online article, 2017). Other symptoms and problems include excessive worrying, panic attacks, anxiety, depression, low self-esteem, risk of drug or alcohol abuse in later teenage and adult life, agoraphobia, social anxiety and claustrophobia.

If left untreated these symptoms can lead to the need for psychotherapy and medication. I personally feel that the link between the rise in mental health problems correlates to symptoms of separation syndrome. Proof of this could be seen in the contrast between rising mental health figures in the developed West compared to fewer cases in the developing East. Where the East has developed and embraced a Western style education system we can see an increase in mental health problems, India and China being two obvious examples.

The need for both parents to work due to economic imperatives means that children spend little time with their family. I know it is not easy to have one parent at home full-time, but the time we do have at home should be utilized to form a strong family bond. Time in the pubs or with friends doing other pursuits means children feeling undervalued. The babysitter, nanny or au-pair can never replace a biological parent. **Note: extra marital affairs with au-pairs and babysitters have ended thousands if not millions of marriages. I know of two cases myself.** This is a risk you take when employing a young woman and allowing her to stay or live in your family home. It would seem that for many couples earning more money has become more important than their marriage and children.

Economic development is termed "progress", however I do not see it as being anything other than a regressive phase for humanity. Whilst we amass material and monetary wealth our children remain locked up in kindergartens, schools and university halls, and let us not forget those that end up in prison.

This may or may not be related, but 1 in 5 American female college students have been sexually assaulted. (Source: U.S. Justice Department, 2018). What kind of "men" arc wc raising? There have also been over 7000 child-on-child sexual assaults in UK schools from 2009 to 2017. You can do an online search for latest figures.

It is an undisputed fact that most young male offenders in prison did not have or do not have a good male role model. The absent father may have been absent even before the child's birth. We know that an Alpha Male is important in any household, or a boy will assert himself once he reaches puberty. I am not saying that a female parent cannot control or discipline a boy; I am looking at the statistics here, and the reality on the ground. Boys need a father figure. Period.

Absent fathers are a big problem in the United Kingdom and America, and this is linked to a rise in criminal behaviour. An absent father is the most extreme form of Repetitive Separation Syndrome. It is sadly permanent in many cases. The children often do not know if they will ever see the absent parent again. Their father may be in jail or have moved to another town or country. I know some women who refuse to let the father of their children see them, for no reason other than spite and bitterness over a failed marriage or relationship. This is child abuse as far as I am concerned, but the courts cannot do anything to force a woman to cooperate. Many men cannot afford to go to court, which is why organizations such as 'Fathers For Justice' have been formed to help and support them. Parents really need to cooperate for their children's sake and stop being so selfish.

The cutting of emotional ties means there is nothing to keep children at home once they hit puberty. The United Kingdom has the highest number of teenage pregnancies in Europe. I think in part that the girls are looking for the love, attention and ideal family life they were denied as children.

Those children who remain focused on education and career will eventually leave for university; find a job abroad, some will move as far away as Australia or America. The familial bond is no longer a factor in keeping young adults close to home. They have become 'emotional orphans' and feel no emotional ties to home, friends or family. Their elderly parents will inevitably end up in a care home. It is they who will cry for their children, not knowing when they will come to see them again. Is this a case of karma coming full circle?

I do wonder what future our current generation of children will inherit. The luxury of having a traditional family with both parents in a union of marriage is becoming a thing of the past.

STD Dubai

For several years now I have been hearing about HIV/AIDS becoming widespread in the Middle East and Far East. AIDS is a huge problem in nations such as America, Thailand, India, and South Africa where the disease is spread through promiscuous sex, prostitution and the sex industry. Other causes include a lack of good hygiene, poor healthcare, and drug use via shared syringes. I am aware that HIV/AIDS can be contracted through non-sexual acts so please do not think that I am in any way attacking those with HIV/AIDS, my intention here is to help educate people and prevent the disease from spreading, and for those infected to seek help and not infect others.

What I am alarmed by most of all is the number of migrant workers from India, Pakistan and Bangladesh that contract the disease in the United Arab Emirates. So what is going on in the region to have caused this sudden epidemic? I recently spoke to a relative of mine who had secured a very good job in Dubai; a transcript of our conversation is below:

WA: I'm really pleased for you, but you've got to be careful out there as a single man.
R: Don't worry; I'll look after myself.
WA: I know you will, but as a single man you'll face many temptations.

R: Well I don't drink or do drugs so I should be okay.
WA: I was thinking more about women, or rather prostitutes.
R: Oh, right.
WA: You do know there's a big prostitution problem in the UAE?
R: Don't worry, my boss has already warned us.
WA: Really?
R: Yes, he's told us about the AIDS problem out here too.
WA: Well I'm glad to hear that. You just stick around people like him.
R: I intend to.

The number of migrant workers living in the UAE apparently caused this AIDS epidemic. These workers live away from their families for long periods of time and seek sexual pleasure through illegal means such as prostitution. It is common knowledge that Dubai has a huge number of prostitutes working under their pimps. They can be from Russian, Thai, Eastern European and even British and American origin.

HIV/AIDS testing and awareness of the disease has yet to be implemented fully within the UAE, and this has left most people ignorant to the causes and means of preventing the disease. Many still believe that HIV can be transmitted via touching a person with the disease or sharing a toilet. The UAE population is very well educated in general, with 80% going on to higher education, but they have little or no knowledge of HIV/AIDS prevention.

In recent years a programme has began to scan foreign workers for the virus, and if found to have the virus are deported back to their own country. Migrant workers are also tested upon entering the UAE to prevent the disease spreading among the population. However it is unlikely that any HIV positive worker will inform their family and may go on to infect their partners or future partners. You might think that I am exaggerating; but I have been told this by a friend of mine who happens to be a medical doctor of Pakistani origin. He has told me that such cases are being reported in Pakistan. Men are knowingly infecting their partners with the disease. I think such men should be sentenced to life in jail for premeditated manslaughter. Their behaviour is worse than animals.

The Middle East is now amongst the top two regions in the world with the fastest HIV outbreak. This is due to the change in cultural and religious values. Sex outside of marriage for example is one factor (Islam forbids sex outside marriage). Awareness and educational programmes are being rolled out but they come too late for many. Those who do access this new information aren't guaranteed to change their sexual behaviour. Families and communities must work together to raise awareness and warn their children (especially those not married) of the dangers posed by sexually transmitted diseases. Other diseases such as Hepatitis B and Tuberculosis are also on the increase.

The World Health Organisation estimated that 2300 people might be living with HIV/AIDS in the UAE. The exact figures are not available. Recently a 19-year-old girl infected with AIDS was arrested for sleeping with many men knowing she has the virus. She told the police that she wanted to infect as many men as possible as revenge for the man who infected her. I imagine there are men out there doing the same thing, infecting many women in retaliation for their catching the disease from a female partner, lover or prostitute. Male prostitutes are available for men and women; both men and women are spreading the disease. I am not blaming women who I know are being exploited (often by force) by male handlers or traffickers

A good friend of mine from Nigeria has currently completed her PhD in infectious diseases. Her main area of research was on sexually transmitted diseases. I was shocked to hear her tell me about a friend of hers who had contracted HIV from her HIV positive boyfriend. The boyfriend knew he had the disease and was on medication. He deliberately passed on the disease to his girlfriend. She had no idea he had the virus as he had kept this from her during their long-term relationship. My Nigerian friend told me: "Young girls and women are so naive. They just think that the contraceptive pill will stop them getting pregnant, but it won't stop them catching sexually transmitted diseases." How can young women be so naïve?

My Nigerian friend being a Baptist Christian does not have sexual relationships outside of marriage, like me, she also believes that sex should only occur within marriage. This advice could have saved her friend and the boyfriend.

In South Africa things are very bad with around six million people infected with HIV/AIDS. The main cause of the spread of sexually transmitted diseases is a promiscuous society. In the UK there has been a 200% percent increase in sexually transmitted diseases since 1997. Can you see a pattern here? There is definitely a correlation between STDs and promiscuity. 67% of all new cases of HIV/AIDS occur within the homosexual community. Why are people not being warned about such health risks?

I am sure there will be some people on the 'politically correct' and 'liberal' bandwagon who will have issues with this article, and that's fine, they are entitled to their own opinions. I will continue to promote the 'prevention is better than cure' method however; not having sex outside of marriage will always be the best means of saving oneself from such diseases.

I also encourage young men and women who are planning on getting married to have an STD test done before consummating their marriage or before planning to have children. If you live in the West you will know that it is common for men and women to have many boyfriends and girlfriends before getting married. I'm not saying this is right, only that it's better to get checked before settling down. It's just a simple blood test and takes around twenty minutes out of your day.

I will mention this final case that was told to me by a family friend. A guy from the UK married a girl from Pakistan, he later found out that he had HIV, but by then he'd passed it on to his innocent wife. You see, many young men here in the UK sleep around, some with escorts and prostitutes. Some Asian parents will often allow their young sons to sow their wild oats before, and even after getting married. I pity the woman they end up with. It's a life of hell and often ends in tragedy.

The guy can be from abroad too so make sure you get him to have a STD check before you marry him to your daughter in the UK. The idea that people are 'pure' and 'innocent' sadly no longer applies. People are putting themselves at risk of STDs.

India, Pakistan and Bangladesh (prostitution is legal in Bangladesh and India) have many brothels among a thriving sex industry, the women that work there are usually forced into prostitution. Many are trafficked and even kidnapped from villages. There is also a big STD problem in these brothels yet the respective governments and health officials do little or nothing to monitor or shut them down. They are even frequented by some police, local officials and married men. In fact it is common knowledge that many users of prostitution are married men, both in the East and here in the West. So what about those single men who end up marrying your daughter?

An Indian friend of mine recently told me that it is now common practice for Indian men and women to take an STD test before marriage. This action is being taken due to the increase in HIV/AIDS and prostitution. Many of the men that contract HIV/AIDS through prostitution have college degrees.

In Malaysia, some men will have slept with up to fifty prostitutes before getting married. A good Malaysian friend who I can trust gave this information to me. He also told me that even in his conservative nation, sex outside of marriage is common between boyfriend and girlfriend.

We must educate our boys and girls about the vile nature of casual sex and prostitution, its victims and the risks involved. Only by ending the demand for this business can we eradicate it and give women the respect they deserve.

The only way we can help reduce and end HIV/AIDS is to prevent the disease spreading by providing teenagers with sex education and preventing promiscuous sex, marital affairs, drug use and prostitution.

We now live in a time where children are being born with the HIV virus or addicted to cocaine. What have they done to deserve this? Please think about yourself and your loved ones. It's just not worth the risk. I mean is sex really worth dying for? Is such behaviour not like that of animals? Actually, I'd say it is worse than animals. Many people are controlled by lust and desire. They don't care who they harm or kill.

Women (and some men) are seen as objects of sexual gratification. They live a life driven by primal desires. It is no wonder that so many men are being expelled from the UAE, and rightly so. We need to bring back the gentleman and gentlewoman. We must strive to take back the moral high ground.

Take care out there and protect your sexual health.

<u>The Dangers of Porn</u>

'I control my desires; my desires do not control me.'

From John F. Kennedy, to Bill Clinton to Donald Trump you will find a trail of sexual promiscuity. Of course there have been hundreds of other notable individuals that have been involved in extra-marital affairs, Tiger Woods for instance, and then there's the latest from Hollywood's film industry, Harvey Weinstein and U.S. congressman Anthony Weiner being the most talked about. Weiner was jailed recently for 'sexting' a fifteen-year-old girl. After the exposure of sexual abuse in Hollywood dozens of women have come forward to talk about their life changing experiences at the hands of vile individuals such as Weinstein and Weiner. Weiner's wife, Huma Abedin, former aide to then Democratic presidential candidate Hillary Clinton, initially stood by Weiner but eventually announced she was leaving her husband over the scandal. British and French MPs and leaders are not free of extra marital affairs either; you can do an online search and find many that have been unfaithful to their partners. Many have kept mistresses too.

It has been estimated that the viewing of pornography is linked to 20% of all divorce cases. I once knew a lady who told me that her husband was addicted to porn, and that he would even watch it in front of their teenage children. This was the reason she left him. Sadly this won't be the only case of divorce by porn. Let me give you some alarming statistics before I continue on this subject.

- 29,000 people watch pornography per second
- 68 million searches for porn per day

- 160,000 searches for child porn per each day
- A new pornographic site is created every 39 minutes
- Americans spend $1 billion per year on porn
- $1 million is spent on porn per day worldwide
- The U.S.A is the biggest creator of porn. 38,000 new sites are created each year

These figures will give you an idea of how big the problem of porn really is, and how much of a danger it poses to our children and us. Porn is easily downloaded to laptops, smartphones and tablets, etc. Children are now sharing porn at school. Many exchange nude 'selfies', especially girls. There are children as young as eight years old receiving porn links via their 'Junk Mail' folder. How many parents warn their children of such dangers?

The porn problem is widespread, from the rich to poor, black to white, religious and non-religious. Porn affects everybody in every nation and in every society. Imagine if we spent those billions on education, healthcare and homes?

So how does this culture of porn affect the rest of us? Well, like Tiger Woods and Anthony Weiner, you too could end up destroying your marriage, as it is common knowledge that watching of porn leads to affairs and marital break-up. Even if there is no affair the couple's sex life suffers and this too can lead to a separation and divorce. Watching porn is also detrimental to mental and physical health. It can also lead to men becoming impotent and infertile. Their partners may no longer arouse them as they have become addicted to porn. What about the dangers to children? Might a parent go on to sexually abuse his or her own child? It is certainly not uncommon.

The proliferation of pornography has become rampant across the developing world, especially in India and Pakistan. In India there is a rape crisis, with over: '24,923 rapes reported in 2012. Out of these, 24,470 were committed by someone known to the victim (98% of the cases). (Source: National Crime Records Bureau (NCRB) 2013 annual report). India is now sentencing rapists to death, something I hope will help bring an end to this horrific rape crisis.

In Pakistan, child abuse is rampant, especially in so-called "religious" schools. Both India and Pakistan also employ child labour, which leads to further child abuse and sexual exploitation. The very cultural and conservative fabric of these nations are being destroyed by the evils of porn, and Bollywood isn't helping this demise, employing scantily clad women and even porn actresses to "star" in their movies. This is a clear sign that the current batch of film directors have been influenced by porn and are catering for their audience of largely teenage boys and men in their early to late twenties. How will these young men go on to view women? There seems to be no moral compass in the film industry.

This trend in viewing women as sexual objects for the gratification of men is spreading further East, to Malaysia, Indonesia, China and Japan. Rapes and incidents of sexual abuse are on the increase. Paedophilia is a big problem in nations such as Japan and Thailand, increasing largely due to a Western demand for young boys and girls. Children are no longer being protected against sexual predators; who are given lenient sentences and go on to repeat offend. Such offenders are known to be watchers of porn, and who go on to watch more extreme forms and eventually child porn.

A worldwide effort is needed to jail such heinous criminals and end their networks. There should be a war on porn before our societies are morally and spiritually destroyed. With our current leaders I do not see any change happening anytime soon. Even some British MPs have been caught buying porn. Porn is no longer seen as immoral; apparently it's something we all like. It says a lot about our societies.

The dangers to health include numerous sexually transmitted diseases, many of which can cause a woman to become infertile, and suffer life long discomfort. Even condoms do not protect you 100%. Oral sex is the biggest cause of sexually transmitted diseases. In the UK last year (2017) there were over 400,000-recorded STDs. This figure only accounts for those people that bothered to get tested. Women that take the contraceptive pill do not think about STDs. Their boyfriend or other "partners" usually pressure them into not using protection.

We live in a time of 'open relationships' and having multiple partners. The UK has the highest number of teenage pregnancies in Europe. Girls are becoming sexually active much younger than before. Men will want to film and photograph themselves and share the images online, often resulting in girls being bullied and even committing suicide. In many parts of the world, women are being bred and treat like animals. They are being shared among many men; even married couples are engaged in this immoral behaviour.

Here's some sexual health information I found online: 'The watching of pornography increases the risk of sexually transmitted diseases, as it introduces children and teenagers to risky sexual acts, such as oral and anal sex. Oral sex is the most common means of catching infections and diseases: 'Oral sex is the stimulation of the genitals using the mouth and tongue. It is one of the ways that sexually transmitted infections (STIs) are most frequently passed on. You can catch an STI if you have just one sexual partner. However, the more partners you have, the greater the risk of catching an infection' (Source: NHS Choices online, 2018).

These STIs include: gonorrhoea, genital herpes and syphilis. The infections commonly caught through oral sex include Chlamydia, HIV, hepatitis A, hepatitis B, and hepatitis C, genital warts and pubic lice. Remember that condoms do not protect you 100% from such infections and diseases.

This is a very dangerous age in which to be seeking a relationship. Make sure you and your partner get an STD check, especially if you plan on getting married and before having children. You should also insist on not being filmed in the bedroom, as those "films", as we all know through leaked 'sex tapes', will be circulated in schools, colleges and online. Your life and career may be over before you've even graduated. Think before you act in your own 'sex film'. Sexual intimacy between partners, it is not to be shared as a spectator sport, your partner does not respect you or your body if he or she wishes to film such intimacy. He or she is probably addicted to watching pornography, and it should send your alarm bells ringing.

<u>You Can't Tell Me What To Do!</u>

Individualism has been defined as: 'the habit or principle of being independent and self-reliant - a culture that celebrates individualism and wealth.' Another definition is: 'the moral stance, political philosophy, ideology, or social outlook that emphasizes the moral worth of the individual.'

This all sounds fine and well, but has individualism gone too far? Can none of us tell anyone else what to do? It certainly seems to be the case. A lot of children are certainly telling their teachers and parents that they can't tell them what to do. Husbands, wives, partners, children to their elder siblings, etc. none can tell the other what to do. This situation is becoming farcical. Soon we'll have criminals telling the police that they can't tell them what to do, hang on a minute, some of them already do, including child criminals (minors). 'You can't tell me what to do (I have rights)' seems to be the 'get out' card for many. Let's look at the reality and consequences of this 'You can't tell me what to do' attitude.

So, we'll begin with the children. Have you ever heard a child say to their teacher or parent 'You can't tell me what to do?' Ah, the little darlings, where did we go wrong? Teaching has officially become the most stressful of professions (parenting too I'd say) in the

UK. Is it any wonder? You can't even restrain a child without being accused of physical abuse. Restraining a violent child nowadays entails circling them (a teacher's mental energy will keep them at bay) in order to stop them from harming themselves or others.

There have been several cases in UK schools of teachers being beaten, stabbed and even killed by children aged under sixteen. This won't come as a surprise to most of you, but it will shock readers in Asia, Arabia, Africa and the Far East, where teachers are still revered and highly respected. In such nations they are seen as equal to a child's parents and are honoured by the wider community. Teaching used to be a calling for many, sadly nowadays many leave the profession within 2-3 years of securing their first teaching job, many choose to teach abroad in the aforementioned continents. Hearing 'You can't tell me what to do' gets tiring after a few years.

Moving on to adult relationships. Husband says "You can't tell me what to do!" wife says "You can't tell me what to do!" Husband's parents say "You can't tell him what to do!" Wife's brother says, "You can't tell her what to do!" Husband and wife's children say, "You can't tell us what to do!"

What on earth is going on here? You know what, no one can tell any of you what to do! Let's be free to do what ever we like! Let's enjoy total anarchy!

And relax - rant over. So, you can see the absurdity of the above situation. People no longer respect personal boundaries, or the roles of individuals; they step on other people's toes all the time. Marriages are breaking down due to the stubbornness of such individuals. I've heard of dozens of cases within my own social circle. The husband and wife, and their extended families, won't back down or change their mind over some decision made by the husband or wife, and before you know it, all hell has broke loose. The couple separate, the devils (from both families) advise the husband and wife separately, making sure that they remain stubborn and stand their ground. You can guess the outcome. Divorce. No one can tell them what to do now! Unless it's the mother, father, brother, uncle, etc.

No one is really 'free' or 'independent', as someone will always tell us what to do, such as a mother or father telling their children what to do (for their own good, safety, etc). Employers will tell their employees what to do, council staff, police, social workers, doctors, etc. they all tell their clients what to do, and failure to do as they say usually spells disaster.

Imagine if your doctor gave you some advice and you told him or her 'You can't tell me what to do!' 'Fine, go and die an early death.' he'd probably think. This is the same death that occurs with marriage, it dies early thanks to the 'You can't tell me what to do!' attitude. Imagine if we told our boss 'You can't tell me what to do!' 'You're fired!' he'd say. 'Enjoy your independence.' The fact is that we are all dependent on others, be it family, friends, employers, etc.

Someone has to have the final say in a relationship. You can't have two bosses in one company or institute. We can look at the working set-up within a business as a good example. If there are two partners, one will own 49% of the business and the other will own 51%. The reason for this is that when both parties can't agree on a business decision, the one owning 51% of the business will have the final say after consultation. If this is how a business dilemma can be remedied what about a marriage? Surely a marriage is more valuable, more sacred than a business? Have we become so ignorant and proud?

The workings of a business, no matter how important, can never be more important than a couple's marriage. It is for this reason that a husband and wife must agree to allow one partner to have the final say in matters on which they can't agree. It is best to agree to this before marriage. Marriage is based on compromise, thoughtfulness and respect. If both partners can maintain these things (free of extended family interference) then there is no reason why their marriage can't be a success, despite having many differences of opinion. I see too many couples splitting up over the most ridiculous and selfish of reasons, below are some of the examples I have come across:

Wife says her husband doesn't get along with her family, husband says wife doesn't get along with his family, wife wants to work, husband doesn't want his wife working, husband works too much, husband doesn't work enough, wife is too independent, husband is too religious, husband isn't religious enough, wife isn't religious, in-laws always interfere in the marriage, in-laws override the husband or wife's decisions, children don't listen to their mother or father, children are too unruly, husband never takes his wife out, wife doesn't want to go out, has no interests, mental health problems such as depression for which no treatment is sought (some people still think that mental health problems brings shame on the individual or family), the husband is impatient, is a bad father/husband (apparently), doesn't spend enough money on his kids, wife's spending habits are out of control, father wants to 'home school' their children, wife is against it, not enough holidays abroad, bored of married life, etc. None of these 'reasons' warrant a separation or divorce in my opinion.

So, back to individualism (the ideology that we can live free of others), we all know this is complete rubbish. Individualism was merely created by the Capitalist and consumer driven agenda by the elite in order that we consume more. The corporations would rather sell us one of every appliance than have us share between two. We each have one home, one kettle, one fridge, one bed, one cooker, one car, one sink, one microwave, etc. You can see the bigger picture, and it means lots of profit for the corporations that feed us this 'Individualism' on a daily basis. Their slogan should be "Don't let anyone tell you what to do - live alone". Imagine how much money the pharmaceutical companies are making at the expense of our living alone?

So, the next time you think about saying 'You can't tell me what to do!' please stop and think for a moment as to who will really lose out. None of us are really 'independent', we are, and always will be social creatures that rely on others for our physical, emotional and spiritual needs.

Learn to compromise.

The Chapters of Life

The school holidays are upon us, and it has got me thinking about the time I had spent working in schools, but also my own school days and the people I said 'hello' and 'goodbye' to. I am grateful to the friends I had who gave me so much fun in childhood.

Each year we live is a layer of life, like a layer of sediment upon our fertile mind. Just as archaeologists dig through the layers of earth to reveal the earth's past, we too can dig through the yearly layers of our lives and find our past. Every year we live adds a layer of events and experience in the emotional and physical sense. These 'layers' might be a fond memory or an emotional scar we gained whilst on a great adventure.

In these times of war, sectarianism, nationalism, racism and political differences, it becomes even more important that we unite on what we have in common, as the late MP Jo Cox once said. She was an example of a kind soul that could see past our differences.

It does not matter how different we are, violence and abuse should never be used on others. We need to look at one another with compassion, empathy and kindness. Everyone is struggling with his or her own demons, no one has it easy, not even those we think of as 'having it good'. Value one another as part of one family, as one race, the human race. Do not be divided among yourselves.

We all reach a point in life where we realize that everyone and everything matters, that it all makes up who we are. I liken all the people I have met to chapters of a book, a book called 'Life'. This book of Life is full of friends, teachers, builders, family, people of faith and no faith, the white, the black and the brown, the rich and the poor, the educated and uneducated, the tall and the short, the fashionable and the pragmatic, the artist and the film-maker, the taxi driver and the chef, the doctor and the nurse, the vegetarian and the meat lover, and so many more people that I have yet to meet on reading that next chapter.

We must not 'tolerate' each other; we must 'accept' one another. I can tolerate someone smoking, yes, but 'tolerate' is the wrong term to use for someone of another faith or colour.

We all want to live and work in peace. We all want a nice home, a good job and financial security. Let us accept one another as humans, as one race and as one family. Peace.

From Chrysalis to Butterfly

I have been wondering of late on the beauty of four fine butterfly wings. What I wonder at most is the butterfly's chrysalis, the stage of a butterfly between being a larva and an adult. The hard, protective covering of the chrysalis reminds me of how we form our own, hard, protective covering, often through tough times. We have to become 'thick skinned' to survive this life, or form a protective 'wall' or 'front'. Just like the chrysalis of a caterpillar, we too develop behind our layer of protection, our own darkness, only to emerge later as a more beautiful creature.

I liken myself to the caterpillar when going through creative or difficult times, as I know that I too will form a *metaphorical* chrysalis and will reappear again. I once read somewhere that we change every seven years, that we become a new person. I have been thinking about how different I was at seven, fourteen, twenty-one and so on, and how I changed during those years. I think there is some truth in the seven years theory; at least I feel there is for me.

We all need to hide away from the world at times, but this does not mean we are lost or defeated, it just means we are growing stronger internally. You will survive a divorce, a bereavement, financial loss, etc. You managed in life before you were married, before you lost all that money or your job. You have everything you need to survive and become stronger. Never give up. You can make it through the trials of life. I have yet to meet anyone that has had it easy; most of the people, if not all of the people I meet, have or have had major challenges in life. Many have lost loved ones, businesses, good health, etc. The one thing they all have in common however is that they refused to give up on life; they have strived to get back on their feet and move on. They might not be as wealthy as before, or wear the fine clothes they once had, but they are content.

This life is but a fleeting shadow, from cradle to grave, it will pass before you know it. Forty-three years of my life have been spent, and God alone knows how long I will live. I still feel like I am twenty-two, that may school and college days weren't so long ago, and that the friends I had made still live nearby. I like to think I have lived a good life so far, and that I am capable of doing more good. I don't think I have upset or hurt anyone intentionally, and hope that I never will. We must make the most of our birth before death, youth before old age, and health before illness.

I hope that what I have shared with you will make you see the bigger picture of life. How you are just one pixel in a greater image. How we all matter and how we can all be a part of a successful community, nation and world. Your one good act of kindness really can change your life and the lives of those around you.

I hope you will be able to relate to my life so far, and to the caterpillar and seven year theory. I hope that you will see how we all have to crawl and climb initially, but have the potential to soar like a butterfly.

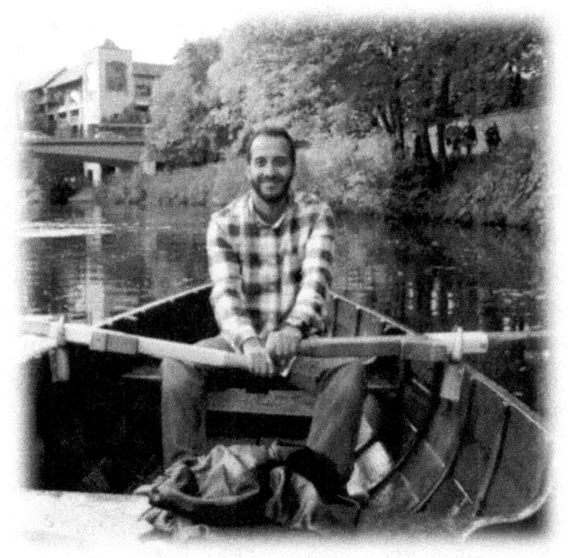

Wishing you a life of wellbeing.

-W. M. Aslam
February 2018

More books by W. M. Aslam

Fiction

Toby Glass and the Terracotta Army
Dawn – the girl who speaks to ghosts
The Life and Death of Danny McGhee
Scott McNally's Mystery
The Very Strange Tale of Mr. Straw
Beneath My Bed
Four Charming Tales For Children

Poetry

Eastern Heart Vocabulary
Open Heart Vocabulary
Graphic Heart Vocabulary
Rhyming Vice
Childsworth
Fifteen Decibel